The New Hot

Taking on the Menopause with Attitude and Style

Meg Mathews

Vermilion
LONDON

This book is dedicated to:

Anaïs, the light of my life

My dad for being Stan the Man

My mum who would have been so proud to see what I am doing

Oscar (RIP) and Ziggy for spending hours with me when I was filled with anxiety

Neeley Moore, my soul sister

Pippy la la for my morning phone calls

Caroline Alexander-Cheong for believing in me

Dr Tiago Justo for all your patience

Steve Hyde thank you for believing in MM

And everyone who keeps me sober – you know who you are…

Contents

FOREWORD

BY DR LOUISE NEWSON, GP AND MENOPAUSE SPECIALIST

Why is this book so essential? Because even I, a GP and menopause specialist, didn't realise at first why I was feeling so off when my menopause happened.

A few years ago, when I was 46, I started to feel more tired than I had ever felt before. My energy levels had reduced and my motivation was much lower than it had ever been. Yes, I was busy. I had recently set up a menopause clinic and was writing content for my My Menopause Doctor website, and yes, I have three daughters, but my life is always busy, so I could see no obvious reason for this sudden overwhelming fatigue. My memory was also worsening – I was finding it much harder to remember even simple things such as where I had left my car keys and the birthdays of friends, but more worryingly I was struggling to remember names of medications at work. I generally felt lower in my mood and less interested in things. My migraines were worsening both in frequency and severity. My joints were stiff and my muscles were sore so I had stopped practising yoga. I presumed all these symptoms were related to working too hard and being pulled in too many directions at work and home.

Although I could hide many of these symptoms from my family, I found I was becoming much more irritable and short-tempered with them. Then one evening, I shouted at one of my teenage daughters because she was late going to bed – she responded by questioning whether I needed to have my period because my mood was so foul! She explained that many of her friends were more irritable and moodier in the days before their periods and I was behaving in a similar way. Then the penny dropped! I realised I had not actually had a period for several months and all of my symptoms were clearly related to being perimenopausal. Despite being a menopause specialist and seeing women with similar symptoms all the time, I had not recognised that my own symptoms had been related to my changing hormone levels.

I know I'm not alone in not recognising my symptoms. The menopause is guaranteed to happen to all women across the globe, yet it is still a taboo to discuss. Most women know few facts about what the menopause means and rarely know about the potential long-term health risks associated with having low hormone levels. Even more worrying is that the majority of doctors and nurses (myself included) do not have any formal training about the menopause as we qualify. It's up to us to educate ourselves later in our career. Now, the majority of what I talk and think about is the menopause, but that isn't the case for all medical professionals.

It took Meg months for her symptoms to be associated with her hormones but there are millions of women worldwide who are never, ever diagnosed correctly. Instead they are misdiagnosed with conditions such as depression, anxiety, fibromyalgia, chronic fatigue syndrome, worsening migraines, cystitis and even dementia.

Meg and I have spent many hours sharing stories and plotting ways of helping such women on a larger scale. Although we laugh a lot together, we also share our feelings of frustration and disappointment that so many women worldwide are still not being given the correct advice or information, despite there being published menopause guidelines from which healthcare professionals should be working.

Women need to be able to make the right choices for them about how they manage their perimenopause and menopause. Many of us stumble across a combination of ways that may include HRT, exercise, nutrition, meditation and good sleep hygiene but we all need to find ways that work to minimise our symptoms and optimise our future health. After all, life expectancy for women has increased over time and for many women, the menopause now lasts for several decades. Even those women who do not have symptoms or whose symptoms have gone still have low levels of hormones in their bodies that can affect their health in later life as low levels of oestrogen are associated with an increased risk of heart disease, osteoporosis, type 2 diabetes, obesity, depression and dementia. We need to be educated about our options to counteract this so we can all enjoy, not just our menopause, but happy and healthy lives far into the future.

That's why I was so thrilled to be asked to write this foreword. This book has the potential to be an amazing resource for women, men, healthcare professionals, children – in fact, anyone who knows a woman – to read, enjoy and learn about this part of life! I hope you enjoy it.

'I see menopause as the start of the next fabulous phase of life as a woman. Now is a time to "tune in" to our bodies and embrace this new chapter.'

KIM CATTRALL, ACTRESS

Introduction

Britpop Queen. That's what they used to call me. In 1997, I was the most written about woman after the Spice Girls and Princess Diana. Hanging out in all the cool places, I socialised all day, all night and often all week! Smoking, drinking, taking drugs... I was a hardcore party girl.

Fast forward a couple of decades and things couldn't be more different. My passion is now MegsMenopause and all the work related to it. I'm teetotal, enjoy a totally plant-based diet and am more likely to be in bed with a cup of warm almond milk than attending the opening of an envelope. I am still awake at 5am, but now it's because I'm out walking my dog not staggering home from the hippest club clutching a bottle of Jack Daniel's.

Would I go back to the hedonistic nineties? Absolutely not! I have no regrets and had an absolute blast (at least the bits I remember!). However, I am now so much happier and more self-accepting, and menopause was my kicker to reassess everything. That's why it frustrates me when it is portrayed as such a terrible time for women. We're led to believe it's the beginning of the end, but trust me, Primrose Hill is the only hill I am over – jogging or walking my dog! Talking to women, I hear such amazing stories of reinvention at menopause; women who set off travelling; launch their own businesses; start new relationships; learn new skills – hearing about them

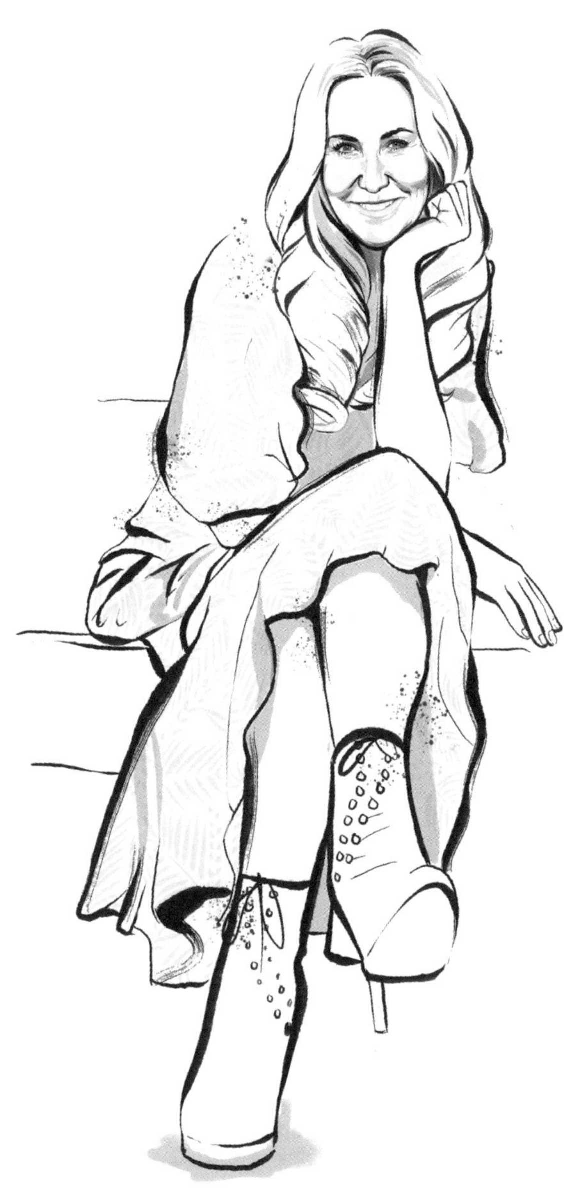

embracing this new chapter in their lives, I can only get more inspired myself.

But it wasn't always a bed of roses. I had a horrendous menopause. Around the age of 47, I came back from a summer holiday and was hit by what I thought was post-holiday blues. Tearful and exhausted, I finally went to the doctor who diagnosed depression and prescribed antidepressants. I took them but I felt awful for the next few years. It was like I was trailing through treacle and wondered if this was it – was this all there was to life?

At the age of 49, I hit an all-time low. Celebrating the New Year with my partner at a lavish country house with great food and an amazing fireworks display, I should have been happy. Miserable and unable to stop crying, I insisted my partner took me home. Social anxiety and depression hit me like a wrecking ball and my life started to fall apart. I got into bed and didn't leave the house for the next three months. I'd always been slim and muscular – now a soft 'menopot' belly was forming as I gained over a stone. Not wanting to bother the doctor, I googled my symptoms. Bad idea. I convinced myself I had a variety of terrible illnesses and diseases. In a very dark place, I was starting to think perhaps I had brought it all on myself with those excesses in my 20s and 30s. Maybe I had fried my brain and my nervous system. My mum had always said my wild ways would catch up with me – was she right?

Approaching 50 was my trigger to tackle how I was feeling. Finally forcing myself out of the house to go to an AA meeting, I hesitantly opened up about how I felt. A wonderful, lovely lady took me to the side and said she thought I might be menopausal. What? I'd always been one of those lucky women who had no period problems. Back at school I never had a day off games or classes unlike friends who had heavy flow or needed to eat six bars of Dairy Milk when their period came. In later life, I found it difficult to relate to women who had PMT and suddenly had the urge to injure their husbands. Even my pregnancy was a breeze – and I was supposed to think my hormones were letting me down now? I resent like hell that I had no idea what perimenopause, menopause and post-menopause were until I was slap bang in the middle of it all.

Armed with more knowledge, I headed to the doctor again and finally got an accurate diagnosis. However, even then I paid to go to a private menopause clinic as the wait for the NHS one was so long, and I could not bear to suffer any longer. It is appalling that so little support is out there for something that will affect half the population. This isn't right and it isn't fair! And I can't help but think that if men hit an age where they suddenly started going off sex, found their penis drying up, and walked about bathed in sweat ready to punch anyone that looked the wrong way at them, things might be very different. Why are there not even stories in the soaps about the menopause? Imagine the conversations that would have been sparked if Bet Lynch had even one hot flush behind the bar at the Rovers Return!

This was the driver for me starting **MegsMenopause.com** and for writing this book. I want to break down the taboos and communicate frankly about the menopause. Not just for menopausal women but also to the significant others in their lives. Like any change, menopause is scary when you don't know how to deal with it. This book is about giving you the knowledge of what to look out for and how to own it.

HOW THE BOOK WORKS

Each chapter tackles a menopausal topic. In each one, I tell you a bit about me in *My Story*: how the menopause affected me and what I have tried to do to alleviate the symptoms.

A word of warning though – I am an addict and will try anything. Absolutely anything! Tapping, acupuncture, working with a healer in Hawaii, using crystals, taking so many vitamins I rattled... I spent thousands in my first year of menopause. Instant gratification was what I was after, trying one thing then moving on.

This is my story and while I make no apologies for it, I am certainly not recommending you follow my path. I am also aware that I am privileged and can afford to try some things that are out of reach to many others.

We then move to the science. I have met a lot of wonderful menopause professionals through this work and many of them appear in this book. I want to thank them for responding so positively when I asked them to put their expertise into each chapter. Their sections will really help explain what's happening to you, why, and what the medical profession can offer to help you. I had to put up with a lot of scolding for my approach as they gave their evidence-based expertise. But hey, I don't mind taking one for the meno team!

One note here – the experts do talk a lot about the positives of HRT. There's a good reason for this as it is the most established and proven way to counteract so many of the symptoms women experience – and protect your health later in life. But, I know that many of you, can't or don't want to take HRT – and that's okay, you can handle menopause without it. In fact, we've got a whole two sections looking at how to tackle the menopause through natural medicine and lifestyle changes.

Each section also contains some *Take Control* tips. These are the best practical suggestions that I, our experts and the rest of the MegsMenopause team have discovered over the last few years to get you through the day dodging whatever meno-missiles get thrown at you. They'll help you get through menopause while you live your daily life – and come out the other side with your sense of self, style and humour fully intact. Right now that might seem like an impossible dream, but it can be done. Trust me.

Lastly, I've included some stories from people I have met over the last few years. Hearing their experiences has been fascinating for me. Nobody used to talk to me – I think I was a bit scary. But now people in the hairdresser chat, attendees at my conferences talk to me, people stop me in the street to tell me their experience – and everyone is different. A huge thanks to everyone who contributed their stories.

I hope that this combination of medical advice, practical tips and personal stories aims to help you feel more empowered about what's happening and how you can handle it. Every single woman is different, what you experience, need and want during menopause will not be the same as me or anyone else, and whatever parts of our advice you use, I hope this book helps support you in your own personal journey.

Happy reading, menos!

With love and sparkle

MEG x

Meg Mathews

'It was at the point that I felt like my life was falling apart around me that I started to ask what could be going on internally, and friends suggested it might be hormonal.'

GILLIAN ANDERSON,
ACTRESS AND AUTHOR

ONE

What The Hell is Going On?

My Story

There is an adage: 'Listen to your body when it whispers because then you won't have to hear it scream.' That sums up menopause to me – not every woman experiences symptoms, while others have a terrible time – but, ignoring what's happening can lead to your body screaming so loud you will finally be forced to listen.

My menopause crept up on me – gently whispering with anxiety and night sweats. Like many women, I ignored the signs. That's one of the things with menopause – it comes when you also have so many other things on your plate. Growing children or teenagers, ageing parents and work compete for our attention and we get pushed down our own to-do list. I was so busy trying to get on with life and be a 'superwoman' who could do it all that my body had to start screaming before I listened to what it was telling me.

I had heard of the menopause, of course, but I didn't really know what it would mean for me. I thought my periods would stop and I might feel hot a couple of times. And it would stop there! I had never heard of 'perimenopause' – the time when your oestrogen levels start to fall and didn't know that you can have menopausal symptoms then – sometimes more severely than once your periods actually stop.

Anxiety was my worse symptom but, as you'll read as the book goes on, there were many more, and I hear countless stories from other women who think they are hypochondriacs as they have been to the doctor so often with symptoms like joint pain; fatigue; night sweats and weight gain round the middle, yet not been given any solutions. Misdiagnosing the menopause costs the NHS millions as people get treated for things like fibromyalgia; migraines; depression; chronic fatigue; and thyroid issues. This happens because there is a real lack of knowledge around the menopause. Trying to find information was very daunting and confusing for me. Maybe it is because it isn't that long since we would have kicked the bucket either before, or not long after, menopause, so it didn't seem worth talking about. But nowadays we are likely to have decades left to enjoy.

The taboo around the topic doesn't help. In 1948, the menopause was mentioned on one radio show and there was a huge outcry – 'lowering of broadcasting standards' and 'acutely embarrassing' were two of the many complaints. And I think that reluctance to talk remains – even now, one TV channel I appear on won't let me use the word – although I am doing all I can to reverse that. In my 'ideal menopausal world', every woman would get a letter or email from the NHS when they are 45 to tell them all about what's going on and what to expect.

Admittedly, it is easy to freak out when you realise what is happening to you. Don't fear the word 'menopause'. It isn't a disease. It is a rite of passage that every woman goes through. I am five years in and there really is light at the end of the tunnel. At the worst times I simply said to myself 'this too will pass' and it did – and I now feel older, wiser and more comfortable in my life than ever.

To get to that point, though, it helps to understand what's happening to your body and why, so over to expert, Dr Laura Jarvis, to explain it . . .

expert view

LET'S TALK ABOUT . . . WHAT'S HAPPENING

WITH DR LAURA JARVIS, MENOPAUSE SPECIALIST AND PSYCHOSEXUAL THERAPIST

I have worked as a menopause specialist for almost 20 years, helping thousands of women in that time, and it's so interesting to me that the menopause transition can be challenging for some, while others seem to cruise through unaffected. It definitely feels a little unfair.

It's not known why women have menopause - most animals are fertile throughout old age. Nor do we know exactly what triggers it. What we do know is that women are born with the total number of eggs they will have for their whole lifetime. Once you reach puberty, the pituitary gland releases hormones (Luteinising Hormone (LH) and Follicle Stimulating Hormone (FSH)) that stimulate the ovaries to release an egg. The ovaries are also what produce most of the oestrogen in the body. As we get older, we lose eggs through ovulation and the ovaries become less responsive to LH and FSH. As a result, the ovaries produce less oestrogen. It's believed this combination is related to triggering menopause - but we're not sure exactly what happens.

WHY DOES MENOPAUSE AFFECT SO MANY THINGS?

Because almost every system in our bodies responds to oestrogen, it's not surprising that the symptoms accompanying its fall are many and varied. The average age of menopause is 51, but there is a large spectrum as to when exactly it occurs, with some women unfortunately experiencing a very early menopause in their early 20s. Exactly why menopause occurs at different ages is also not well understood. We know that, for example, if your mum had a very early menopause it might increase your likelihood of having one too, but even that is not absolutely guaranteed.

SO, WHEN ARE YOU IN MENOPAUSE?

This causes some confusion. The definition of menopause is quite simply the cessation of periods but to be defined as being 'in menopause' you have to have had no periods for at least a year. The perimenopause is the phase leading up to this point. The phase of 'post-menopause' begins after you have had no periods for a year.

The symptoms of the perimenopause and menopause last for four years on average, but once again, this is a huge spectrum with some women experiencing no symptoms at all and some women still having them in their 70s.

Here comes the rub. Menopause often hits women when their teenage kids are kicking off or preparing to leave home; elderly parents are beginning to fail; and grey hair and wrinkles have taken hold. It is not difficult to see that this toxic mix can lead to a 'perfect storm' of problems. So, how do you know if what you're experiencing is the stress of normal life or the effects of your changing hormones? Well, often it can be quite obvious. If somebody comes to me and they say, 'I'm struggling to sleep and I am sweating and flushing' and I say to them, 'When was your last period' and they say, 'oh, it was about six months ago', that will lead me to think that they are menopausal or perimenopausal. Other times it's less clear cut.

SHOULD YOU HAVE YOUR HORMONES MEASURED?

A test for Follicle Stimulating Hormone (FSH), which rises during menopause, is useful for women under the age of 45 years where there is some ambiguity around whether someone is menopausal and they have stopped their periods. But if someone is over 45 years and has stopped their periods, checking their FSH does not provide us with any useful information. The only exception is when someone is using progesterone-only contraception, which may stop their periods. If someone is taking the combined pill, they need to stop for six weeks before an FSH test can be taken. One question I'm often asked is whether women need to see a doctor at the menopause if their symptoms aren't concerning them. My advice is that it is definitely worth having a conversation with your GP to make sure you have good lifestyle advice and information about Hormone Replacement Therapy (HRT) even if you're not sure you're going to use it. I am sometimes frustrated when I see women who should maybe have been offered HRT because they have a family history of osteoporosis, for example, and missed the boat because they didn't have that conversation.

The other reason it's good to chat to your GP is that menopause is the ideal time to stop and take stock of your general life and health. Women now live up to a third of their lives in the menopause so it is important to make sure it is as healthy as possible. Menopause is also a great time to lose that extra

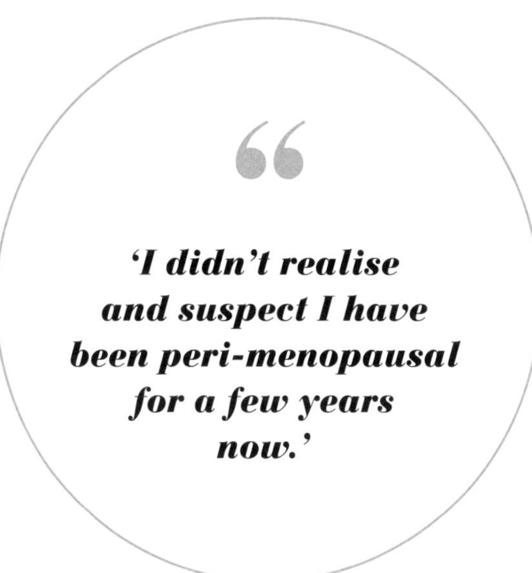

weight you have been planning to shed for a while, to stop smoking or become more active. Make time for yourself and invest in your body (it's the only one you have!).

For some, the menopause has a lot of negative connotations, but I take a slightly different view. Old age is a gift not afforded to everyone, my father included. He died in his early 50s and missed out on so much of life. I am therefore determined to enjoy my post-menopausal years.

My bucket list gets longer by the day; bring it on!

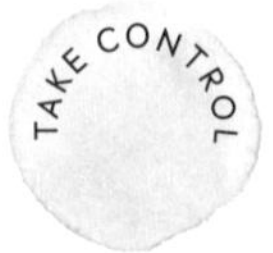

Do a Meno-Audit

These are the most commonly established symptoms of menopause. Knowing how many you are experiencing can give you – and your doctor – a clue as to what's happening. Have a look and see how many you tick off. You may also want to take it to the doctor when you go for your first appointment.

Common Symptoms

- Hot Flushes
- Night Sweats
- Loss of Libido
- Vaginal Dryness
- Irregular Period

Mental Symptoms

- Anxiety
- Irritability
- Panic Disorders
- Difficult Concentrating
- Mood Swings
- Foggy Brain
- Depression

Physical Changes

- Fatigue
- Hair Loss
- Sleep Problems
- Dizziness
- Weight Gain
- Bloating
- Allergies
- Brittle Nails
- Osteoporosis
- Irregular Heartbeat
- Changes in Body Odour
- Bladder Problems

Pains

- Breast Pain
- Headaches
- Joint Pain
- Electric Shock
- Burning Mouth
- Nausea and Digestive Problems
- Dental Problems
- Muscle Tension
- Dry and itchy skin
- Tingling Extremities

Total Number of Symptoms

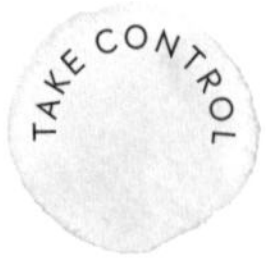

Cervical screening

You may be used to having smear tests every three years, but once you reach 50, the risk of cervical cancer falls and you will only be invited to attend every five years. Yay! Because of changes to the vagina that happen during menopause, tests might get a little bit more uncomfortable now, but we have some tips on page 86 that might help. Cervical screening stops at age 65, unless one of your last three tests was abnormal, when they'll keep monitoring you. You don't need smear tests if you have had a total hysterectomy that removed your womb and cervix.

- **Dental checks**
  The health of your teeth and gums can change after menopause so make sure you see your dentist when your next check is due.

- **Eye tests**
  You should have one of these every two years – more often if you have a family history of glaucoma or have type 2 diabetes.

- **Hearing tests**
  Past 50 it's suggested you have a hearing test every two years or if you notice your hearing is declining. Untreated hearing loss may be linked to the faster progression of some other health problems in later life so it's not something to ignore.

- **NHS Health Check**
  This is offered to adults in England aged 40–74 and is designed to spot early signs of stroke, kidney disease, heart disease, type 2 diabetes and dementia. You'll be invited for a check around your 40th birthday and every five years afterwards.

- **Mammogram**
  This checks your breasts for lumps far smaller than you might feel yourself. Not all lumps found by mammogram are cancerous, but it's important to be screened. You'll be invited for your first mammogram at 50 then again every three years until you're 71.

BENEFITS OF THE MENOPAUSE

No, I haven't made some kind of brain-fog-related typo here - I actually do want to talk about the positive side of menopause. Because there is one - and it's important to know that. Some cultures even look at the menopause as something to look forward to, a time when you develop a status and wisdom you don't have during your younger years. I know this is going to be hard to believe when you're standing there trying not to burst into tears because you've lost your car keys again or every muscle in your body aches, but keeping the positives in mind can help you get through those tough days.

The way I look at it, I'm 52 now (and you're probably about the same age) and I want to live at least into my 80s. Am I supposed to spend all that time feeling bad about the fact that I'm post-menopausal? No way! So, here's a few positives about the menopause to think about:

- No more periods, PMS or cramps.
- Many women get a massive rush of energy and enthusiasm for life post-menopause.
- You'll save money on tampons and pads.
- You'll never ruin your favourite undies again.
- Fibroids shrink and often get better. Endometriosis also disappears.
- Some migraine sufferers find their headaches stop.
- You're still only at the halfway point of your life – the best is yet to come.
- It's a great excuse to take stock and make sure you're happy and make any changes if you're not (you can always blame your hormones).
- Exercise works better now – you actually burn more fat doing it than you did before.
- You don't have to worry about contraception ever again (but obviously still practice safe sex if you're not in a steady relationship). Or, an accidental pregnancy. This can make some women enjoy sex more – hello orgasms!
- Getting through the bad days makes you realise you can do anything. Those bad days are only temporary – and you can get help for them.
- This new phase of life can strengthen your relationship and improve your sex life if you start to talk more.
- You realise you need to put yourself first – we don't do that enough.

'I now play what I call Menopause Bingo with my friends, I share a list of symptoms with a group of women and see who ticks off the most. I played with a group of my friends recently and it was hilarious, we all had something we were dealing with, hot flushes, brain fog, or night sweats but no-one has exactly the same symptoms.

LOUISE MINCHIN,
JOURNALIST & TV PRESENTER

TWO

At War with My Body

My Story

That list of 34 symptoms of menopause you just ticked on page 23 – I had 32 of them. The mental symptoms for me were definitely the worst, but then the physical symptoms came along to join my menopausal party.

The worst was the start of osteoporosis. Osteoporosis translates to 'porous bones' and it leads to weak and brittle ones. A DEXA scan, which effectively measures the strength of your bones, showed my right hip was suffering. Menopause doesn't cause osteoporosis directly; it is caused by a deficiency of calcium in the bones. But oestrogen plays an important role in getting the calcium to your bones. So, as oestrogen levels drop during menopause, the possibility of osteoporosis increases. My mum had osteoporosis and was bedridden for the last few years of her life, so my diagnosis scared the living daylights out of me. My independence is important, and I hate the thought of having to be looked after, but many people who suffer a hip fracture from osteoporosis end up dependent on caregivers. So, I am doing all I can now to protect myself against it getting worse. I cover the steps I am taking in my exercise and nutrition chapters, later in the book, but essentially, with the help of HRT, the right food and exercise and some supplements I have moved my DEXA scan out of the red and it now borders amber/green. I'm working to keep improving it further.

I also developed a dry mouth and waves of nausea – and then I got breast pain. The only time I could remember having breast pain was when I was pregnant with Anaïs. When I then realised I also hadn't had a period in a number of months, a surge of rising panic spread through me and I rushed to the chemist and bought a handful of pregnancy tests. They reassured me I wasn't pregnant – but if I wasn't, what was going on? Turns out breast pain and tenderness are other symptoms I hadn't known were associated with menopause.

Lastly, there was the sleep stuff. My night sweats were a nightmare – having to get up and change myself and the sheets during the night. This added to the menopausal fatigue I was already suffering, making me so tired during the day that I could barely function.

This all sounds fun, doesn't it! But, remember, everyone is different and you may get some, all – or none – of these symptoms, So, the question is: why do all these things happen – and how can you help tackle them? Over to my next expert.

expert view

LET'S TALK ABOUT . . . PHYSICAL SYMPTOMS

WITH DR ANNE HENDERSON, MENOPAUSE SPECIALIST

When I'm lecturing on menopause I describe it as a 'top-to-toe' phenomenon. There's literally not a part of the body that doesn't have some form of oestrogen receptor in it, and considering oestrogen generally has hugely positive effects on the body, it's not surprising that we experience so many negative effects when levels start to fall.

The physical symptoms of menopause can be extremely varied – but we can generally group them into clusters:

THE VASOMOTOR SYMPTOMS

These include hot flushes, night sweats and dizziness and they come from changes in oestrogen receptors in the central nervous system. The classic hot flush is described as the sense of heat rising up from the pit of your stomach, up to your chest and neck, up through the face. And in some women it isn't just a sensation, they can also go bright red, which, for some women, is very embarrassing. Flushes can happen just once a day, but I have patients who struggle with them six to 10 times an hour, day and night.

When flushes occur overnight they are given the term night sweats - and while they can just affect the upper body, you can find you wake up literally drenched all over in sweat, which disturbs sleep - many women report having to get up to change the bedding or bed clothes, or lie on a towel.

One myth about these symptoms is that they are short-lived and you just need to put up with them for a year or so, but up to 15 per cent of women will have vasomotor symptoms for at least five years.

HRT (HORMONE REPLACEMENT THERAPY) is the most effective treatment for these symptoms (there is a blood pressure drug called Clonidine which can help, and SSRI antidepressant drugs like Prozac can be used, but neither should be your first line of treatment as they have pretty major side effects and are not particularly effective).

Lifestyle measures can also make a difference (you'll hear about some herbal solutions and dietary changes later in the book) but also look into specialist menopause clothing made from temperature-regulating fabrics which can help, especially at night.

Vasomotor symptoms can also be associated with a change in body odour. Even if you're not visibly aware of being drenched in sweat, there is usually a higher level of sweat production during menopause and body odour may be associated with that.

Other women notice a change in the odour of their vaginal secretions - this is related to a change in the vaginal pH. Normally this would be very acidic but as oestrogen levels fall, pH rises, and the microbiome (the bacteria that populate the body) gets unbalanced, which changes odour. Good personal hygiene can help, while probiotics might positively alter bacteria balance.

MUSCULOSKELETAL SYMPTOMS

These are part of a cluster of symptoms like pain or muscle tension that involve joints, ligaments , muscles, and basically the whole skeleton. They tend to happen earlier in the menopause, and unfortunately they're very symptomatic. It's a very interesting problem, but one that is not fully understood: falling oestrogen causes collagen depletion that may play a role, but the changing balance between oestrogen and progesterone may also affect receptors in the joints. We do know that unlike joint problems like arthritis, this is not an inflammatory process, so drugs like ibuprofen won't help.

Problems in smaller joints like hands and feet can be hard to tackle without HRT, but where problems are in the larger joints, exercise is an excellent solution, particularly strength training. Exercise also helps offset muscle loss (you can lose more than 2 per cent of muscle mass a year in the run up to menopause), and strengthens the support around the joints.

Flexibility exercises also help lengthen the ligaments and prevent muscle tightness that can also contribute to pain, so I suggest regular stretching. There is also evidence that taking supplements like fish oils containing unsaturated fatty acids may help. Osteoporosis falls into the musculoskeletal group but it's generally symptom-free until late in the disease when women start to develop fractures. Lowering osteoporosis risk is one of the main benefits of taking HRT.

DIGESTIVE SYMPTOMS

These are linked to the change in balance between oestrogen and progesterone that happens at menopause – progesterone acts

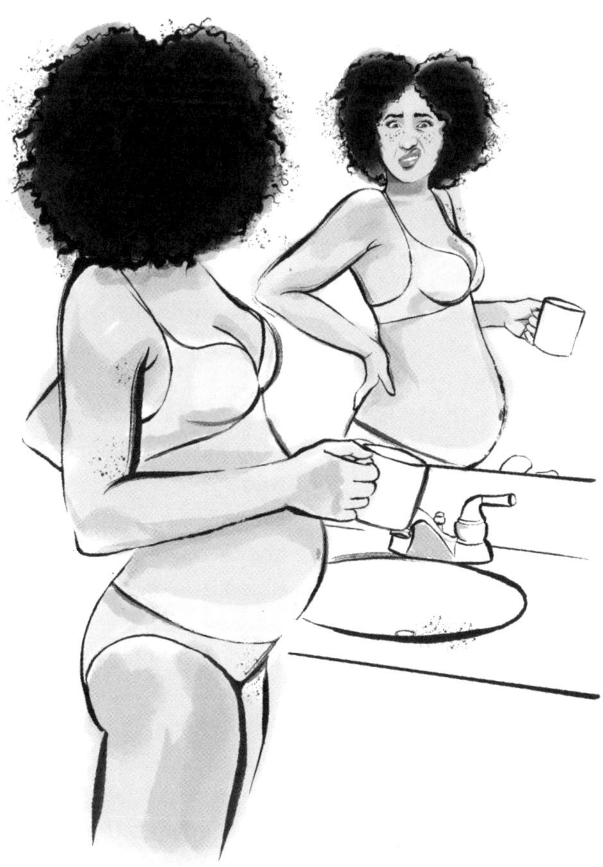

on smooth muscle tissue from which the gut is largely created. You might get an almost IBS-type (Irritable Bowel Syndrome) symptom of constipation along with loose bowel motions. Bloating happens when the gut is sluggish causing it to blow up with contents and gas. This can also lead to nausea.

Good general gut health will help, so look after the gut microbiome with a high-quality probiotic (and look at the tips on page 169), but also consider the content of your diet and see if any food aggravates symptoms. I sometimes recommend my menopausal patients investigate the FODMAP regime which many people with IBS follow to see if it helps.

SENSATION-BASED SYMPTOMS

These can include a feeling of burning in the mouth, tingling extremities, electric shocks and something called 'formication', which is the sensation of ants crawling on the skin. This group of symptoms are much less common than the others that we've discussed, but they can be very difficult to live with. Treating these can be hard as it's likely the feelings are not coming from the skin or mouth itself but are triggered at a central level in the brain.

You can use mouthwash with a local anaesthetic to reduce the symptoms in the mouth, but topical treatments like anti-itch or steroid creams won't work on skin symptoms as it's not a skin complaint.

BREAST PAIN

This symptom, like the problems in the gut, is linked to the fluctuating balance between oestrogen and progesterone, which triggers discomfort. The best ways to manage it without HRT are high doses of unsaturated fatty acids like evening primrose oil and starflower oil and wearing a supportive bra (I suggest patients wear a moderate to high-impact sports bra, not an underwired one, 24/7). The good news is that breast pain does tend to stop when your periods do; it's not usually a symptom that lingers.

There is another cluster of physical symptoms called 'genitourinary syndrome of menopause'. This was something that Meg found hit her particularly hard, so we'll cover those in detail on page 82. If you're now reading this somewhat overwhelmed and worried about what might be in store, remember, almost all of the above can be dealt with – if you just ask for help.

Reducing vaginal odour

Chances are you're the only person who will notice this change, but if this is starting to sap your confidence, here are some tips that help:

1. Wear breathable fabrics like cotton as these are less likely to trap sweat, which can make odour worse.

2. Try a probiotic. A bacteria called Lactobacillus helps keep your vagina pH balanced, so taking a probiotic strain that contains this might help rebalance things.

3. Rinse the vulva area regularly with plain water or a soap-free wash (soap can cause itching and irritation if used too often).

4. Your doctor can prescribe an oestrogen cream which may rebalance the pH

5. If you have other symptoms like itching, burning or changes in discharge, mention these to your doctor just in case it's not just your hormones causing the problems.

The breathing technique that reduces hot flushes

This technique comes from experts at San Francisco State University in the US and it was actually discovered by accident. Dr Erik Pepper was teaching his class a type of deep breathing, and some his older female students noticed their hot flushes decreased (while some younger students got fewer menstrual cramps). He investigated and found other research which showed this breathing technique cut the incidence of flushes by 50 per cent.

So, how do you do it? Here's his technique:

- Imagine that you are holding a baby. Now, with your shoulders relaxed, inhale gently so that your abdomen widens.
- Then, as you exhale, purse your lips, and very gently blow over the baby's hair. Allow your abdomen to narrow as you exhale so the baby's hair barely moves. At the same time imagine you can feel the breath flowing away and past your legs. Smile as you exhale.
- Practise inhaling and exhaling like this when you feel a hot flush starting and you may be able to stop some of them in their tracks.

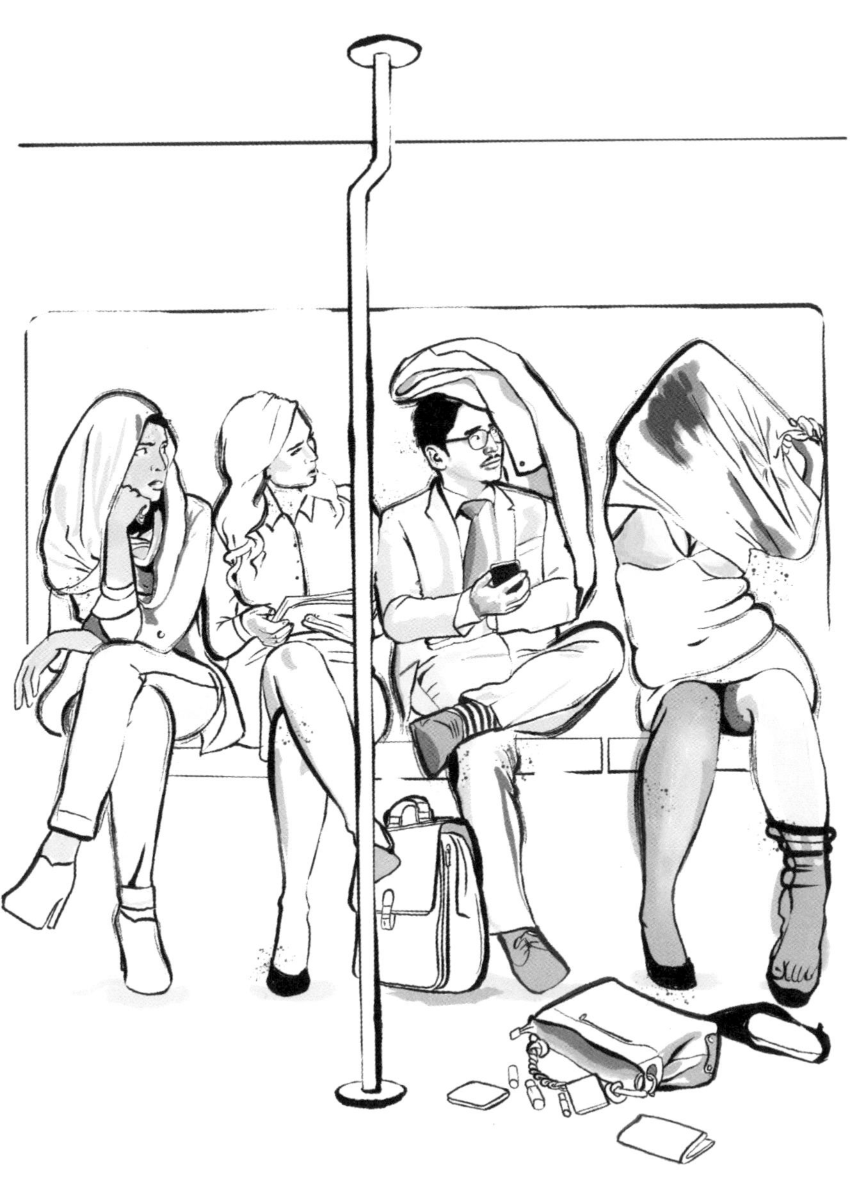

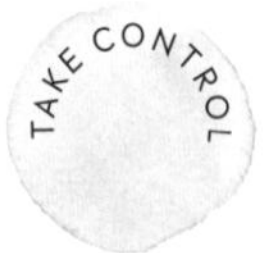

A simple stretching regime to try each day

Staying flexible helps with joint issues, so doing some simple stretches each day can help to alleviate pain. To move your joints through their whole range of motion, personal trainer Christina Howells suggests her clients start their day with the Sun Salutation yoga sequence. This move has many benefits: it is a powerful energiser; it helps release muscular tensions; it stimulates the circulatory and lymphatic systems; and by allowing you to focus on your body and breath, calms the mind. It also boosts your adrenal glands (you'll hear more about those on page 150).

1. Stand up straight, palms of your hands together in front of your chest (as if you are praying). Breathe regularly.

2. Inhale as you raise your arms straight up above your head and carefully bend backwards from the waist a few centimetres until you feel a gentle stretch across your front.

3. Exhale as you bend forwards from your hip joints. Place your hands on the floor either side of your feet (at first you might need to bend your knees to do this but gradually you will become flexible enough to touch the ground with legs straight).

4. Inhale as you look up and step your left foot behind you as far as you can.

5. Step back with your right foot so the weight of your body is balanced on your hands and feet. Your body should now make a straight line from your hands to your feet in a 'plank' position.

6. Exhale as you lower your knees to the floor. Rest your chest then chin on the floor.

7. Inhaling, lower your body so you are lying flat, then slowly arch your back from the waist so your chest comes off the floor. Keep your hands on the floor but your arms will straighten.

8. Exhale, bending your knees, then straighten your arms and legs and push your hips up so you make a V (this is 'downward dog' position).

9. Inhale as you step between your hands with your left foot. Exhale as you step forward with your right foot. Now slowly and while inhaling bring yourself to the standing position.

10. Repeat the sequence from step 2 as many times as you like (it should take five minutes to do 20 sequences once you've worked it all out). Just remember each time to lead with a different foot in steps 4 and 9. The faster you carry out the Sun Salutation the more it will energise you, but make sure you understand how to do all the moves first.

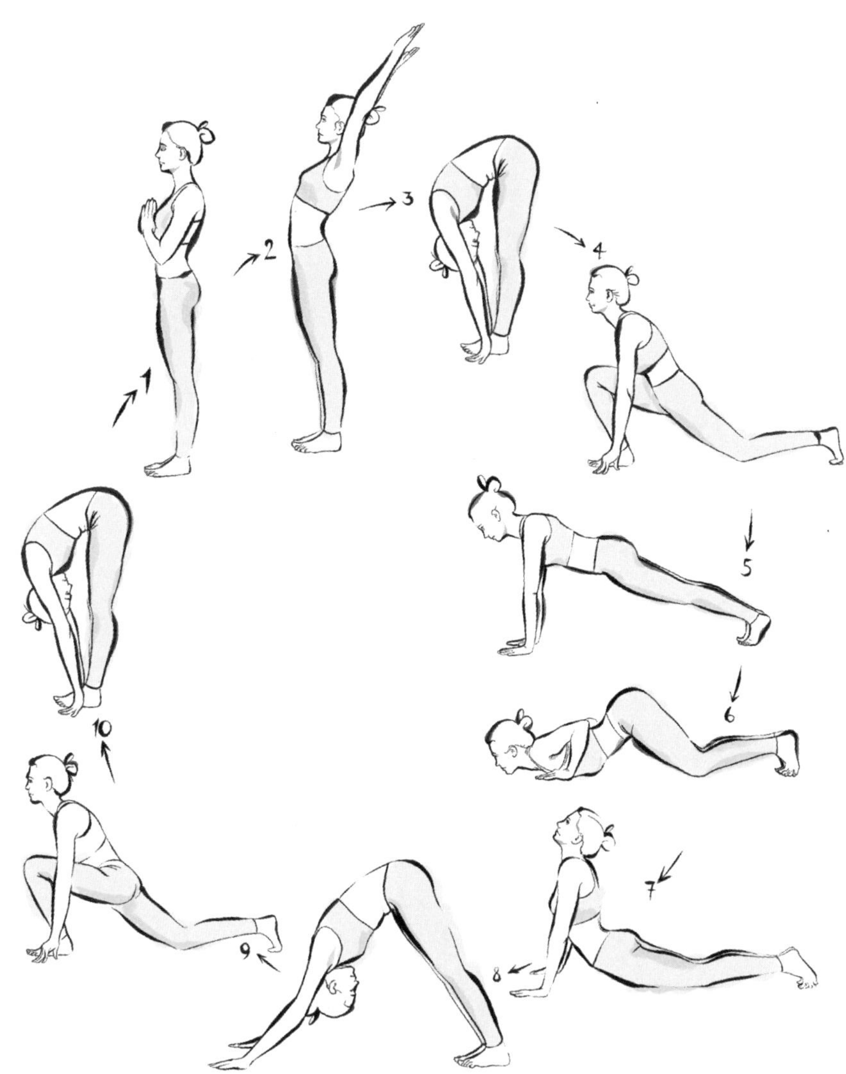
1
2
3
4
5
6
7
8
9
10

WHAT'S A FODMAP DIET?

'FODMAPs' are a group of sugars found in a large number of foods. The name is a shortened version of their full title - Fermentable Oligosaccharides, Disaccharides, Monosaccharides and Polyols. One UK trial showed that avoiding FODMAPs helped 76 per cent of people with IBS reduce their symptoms. This can be helpful to consider if you are experiencing uncomfortable bowel symptoms as part of your menopause.

FODMAPs cause problems when the bacteria that live in the colon use them as food. As this happens, chemicals are produced that can irritate the gut lining and make gas which can trigger symptoms in those with a sensitive gut.

FODMAPs are found in a large number of foods including:

- Anything with wheat in, like bread, pasta, couscous, cakes and biscuits.
- Cow's milk and anything that contains it, like ice cream, cheese and yogurt.
- Some vegetables, including cauliflower, leeks, onions, garlic and mushrooms.
- Some nuts, including pistachios and cashews.
- Some fruits, including apples, apricots, cherries, peaches, pears, prunes and watermelon.
- Some sweeteners, like honey, agave nectar, sorbitol and xylitol.

To find out more, look at *The Complete Low-FODMAP Diet* by Dr Sue Shepherd and Dr Peter Gibson (Vermilion), two leading researchers in the field. They can give you a better idea of what cutting out FODMAPs involves and help you try the diet for a short period to see if it helps. If it does, then it's recommended you see a dietitian, as following a FODMAP-free plan involves cutting out a lot of food groups and it can be hard to balance your diet long-term without professional advice.

'Forgetfulness and fogginess were torture. Sometimes my kids would look at me as if to say . . . who are you? And what have you done with our mother?'

DAVINA MCCALL, TV PRESENTER

THREE

A little bit Crazy

My Story

While I did suffer physical symptoms of menopause, it was the change to my mental health that hit like a tsunami and knocked me off my feet.

I was almost 50 but acting like a hormonal teenager, watching TV in my bedroom all day and night, hiding away from the world. As mentioned in my introduction, at one point I did not leave the house for three months. I was overwhelmed by everything and excited by nothing. Holidays used to be so enjoyable but the thought of packing, getting to the airport and remembering my passport just felt too much. I did make it on holiday to LA once, which should have been amazing, but I spent the whole trip in my hotel bedroom. I was a real fun holiday companion! Christmas was another challenge; I couldn't even be bothered putting a tree up. Diagnosing myself with depression, I took myself to the GP who agreed and gave me antidepressants. Neither of us considered menopause.

I took the antidepressants and felt a little better, but not much. Driving became impossible; I was too anxious and afraid. It was the worst anxiety: the kind with no real root cause. Exhaustion hit me like a truck! Social anxiety then came along to join the party of fatigue and depression and I got to the point where I couldn't even look people in the eye. I used to be out all the time – with a real case of FOMO (*Fear of Missing Out*) when I wasn't – and I loved the company of others, but that stopped overnight as my confidence hit an all-time low. I'd scroll through other people's Facebook posts and feel that everyone else was living their best life – and then there was me. I started to go to a very dark place.

My brain would race and as I suffer from ADHD, I started to worry that it might be getting worse. I was over-emotional and not at all rational. I would sit in trackies and order clothes from the internet that I knew I would never wear. I just could not take a joke; I went ballistic when my partner made a comment about my (lack of) cooking ability. I exploded when my daughter's room was a mess. When I went to a shop and there was a queue, I threw the basket on the floor and marched out. I'm an animal rights activist and if I saw a picture or film with an animal being mistreated it would trigger floods of tears. I started to really miss the person I used to be and wondered if she would ever come back.

When I started having the symptoms in my early 40s, I was still drinking. Self-medicating to try and alleviate them, I would drink more and more, then blame my exhaustion and anxiety on a hangover. I think the perimenopausal symptoms were a factor in my frequent relapses as I started on the path to sobriety.

Things are very different now. I look back at that time as awful, but necessary to get me to where I am now. Free and refreshed is how I would describe myself; others call it 'post-menopausal zest.' A stronger sense of who I am and what I want in life are just two of the benefits of making it to the other side. My FOMO has been replaced with JOMO (Joy of Missing Out). Self-reflection made me realise that I just wanted to be seen in the right places with the right people to feel worthy, so I would hang out with anyone and everyone. But I know now that spending time with quality people is what really makes my heart light up.

So, how did I get there? Well, HRT helped me balance out those pesky hormones and I also use CBD oil to alleviate anxiety. A friend introduced me to it, and from the first time I tried it I found a sense of calm I hadn't felt in a long time. I eased myself off antidepressants as I found myself starting to feel better. That's why I added it to my product range as I was so impressed with its effects; it is important to get the good quality stuff though.

What else helped? Cognitive Behavioural Therapy (CBT). This was part of my rehab and it is all about changing the way you think and behave. I found the exercises useful for getting out of my own head and the 'poor me' mentality I had developed. Online support groups also made me feel a lot less alone. We really are the first generation to start talking about menopause; I dread to think what it must have been like to suffer in silence.

Tattoos with messages that resonated with me also helped. 'Love yourself first' is tattooed down my arm. 'This too will pass' is inked on my chest. Because it does pass.

‘CBT helped me notice my triggers then find ways of working through them – it saved me!’

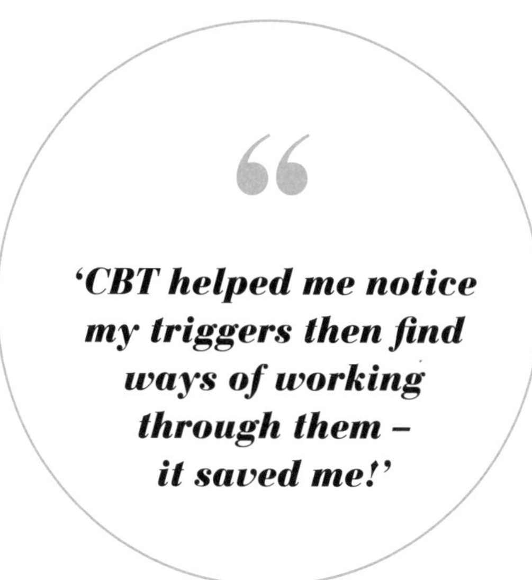

There isn’t an overnight fix, and I still have down days, but they are not so severe or so frequent. You might not want to get tattooed (or maybe you do?) but you could save your positive messages as pop-up reminders on your phone.

Like PMT, some women are lucky and won’t suffer any symptoms as they go through menopause, but if you do (and I’m guessing you probably do if you are reading this book), know that you are not alone and there is help out there. And to talk about it, let’s hand over to two experts in this area. First, Dr Meg Arroll, psychotherapist, who can talk about what the medical profession can offer to fight the mental symptoms of menopause – and then coach Dawn Breslin, who has the most brilliant technique for helping you put yourself first, right now.

expert view

LET'S TALK ABOUT . . . MENOPAUSE & MENTAL HEALTH

WITH DR MEG ARROLL, PSYCHOLOGIST

Psychological and emotional symptoms can be some of the most confusing and frightening aspects of the menopause. Many women ask, 'Am I losing my mind or is it my hormones – and how do I know the difference?' The answer can be complex as physiological processes affect our emotional wellbeing and vice versa.

Depression and anxiety are the two primary mental health issues faced in the menopause. First though, I need to explain that the 'depressed mood' which affects about a third of postmenopausal women, is different from 'clinical depression'. To differentiate, symptoms of clinical depression also include prolonged tiredness, loss of interest in normal activities, weight loss, sadness and irritability alongside that low mood. If you are also experiencing these then you should talk to your GP.

Depression and anxiety often occur together and the symptoms of the latter are characterised by tension, nervousness, panic, worry and feeling on edge. In severe cases, anxiety can lead to panic attacks, causing shortness of breath, chest pain, sweating, dizziness, and heart palpitations - but although panic attacks can be scary and intense, they aren't usually dangerous. They can, however, have a significant the impact on your daily life and functioning.

WHY DOES THE MENOPAUSE LEAD TO ANXIETY AND DEPRESSION?

Oestrogen has many functions, one of which is to calm, so when levels drop, psychological symptoms can be the result. But this isn't the only reason why you might experience emotional symptoms during the menopause. As Dr Jarvis mentioned before, the menopause often happens at exactly the point in your life when you have the most on your plate and the combination of stress and fluctuating hormones can be difficult.

TALKING REALLY CAN HELP

As Meg discovered, one method that can help some of these symptoms is Cognitive Behavioural Therapy (CBT). The theory behind CBT is that we can change our thoughts and beliefs (cognitions) to break behavioural patterns that might be affecting our health. CBT is carried out by a professionally trained therapist over, usually, 6–12 sessions, during which unhelpful thought patterns and behaviours are identified and challenged - for instance, you may think, '*My symptoms are completely ruining my life and I can't do anything properly anymore*,' but the aim of CBT would be to alter this belief so that more supportive thoughts can emerge, such as,

'My symptoms are troublesome at the moment, but I know talking about them with other women will make me feel better'.

Research studies have shown that CBT is a safe treatment, particularly for women who cannot or do not want to use HRT, and it reduces psychological symptoms, improves sleep quality and supports your daily life.

Other talking therapies to consider include hypnotherapy, mindfulness-based stress reduction (MBSR) and relaxation training, all of which have been studied scientifically and shown to help the psychological symptoms of the menopause.

HYPNOTHERAPY

In this treatment, a practitioner will help an individual reach a 'hypnotic state' of deep relaxation, in which health-promoting suggestions are made. You're always in total control over your thoughts and actions; the hypnotherapist merely enables you to focus your attention on inner sensations and experiences. Like CBT, hypnotherapy is safe and doesn't cause the side effects associated with some medications, and research has shown it to be as effective as some drugs for treating menopausal symptoms. Hypnotherapy can also help to improve sleep, concentration and ability to engage in life once again.

MBSR (MINDFULNESS-BASED STRESS REDUCTION)

This is the formal method of mindfulness, which again is taught by a trained practitioner in a course of 6–8 weekly sessions. Mindfulness has become very popular, but it is only these more structured methods that have been studied properly by researchers. MBSR has been found to consistently reduce stress and psychological symptoms in menopausal women.

RELAXATION TRAINING

Relaxation training for menopausal symptoms includes progressive muscle relaxation, slowing down and pacing breathing patterns, and guided imagery. Overall, these techniques appear to reduce general menopausal symptoms, vasomotor symptoms (like hot flushes) and psychological symptoms such as low mood, but should usually be part of a more comprehensive treatment plan. The breath exercise on page 56 is one example of this.

A final word . . .

*Your doctor should take any mental health symptoms you experience seriously. Although it would be a jump too far to say that the menopause leads to suicide, figures from the Office of National Statistics do show that midlife is the time period with the highest rate of suicide in the UK for females between 50 to 54 years. You should feel not only listened to but heard.**

***Source:** *www.ons.gov.uk/peoplepopulationandcommunity/birthsdeathsandmarriages/deaths/bulletins/suicidesintheunitedkingdom/2017registrations#suicide-patterns-by-age*

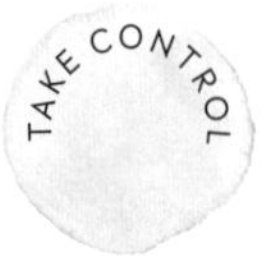

The quick calming exercise to learn

Counsellor Diane Danzebrink has a simple tip to help calm you if you are feeling anxious or overwhelmed:

'One of the first things that I teach my clients with anxiety is to take back control of just one thing in their lives – and, as we all need to breathe, that's often where I like to start. When we breathe out the body can't help but relax, so simply breathing out for longer than we breathe in, with counting in your head, can bring us back to control. Try it. Try breathing in through your nose for a count of one and out from your mouth for a count of three and see how it makes you feel. Use it whenever you start to feel overwhelmed.'

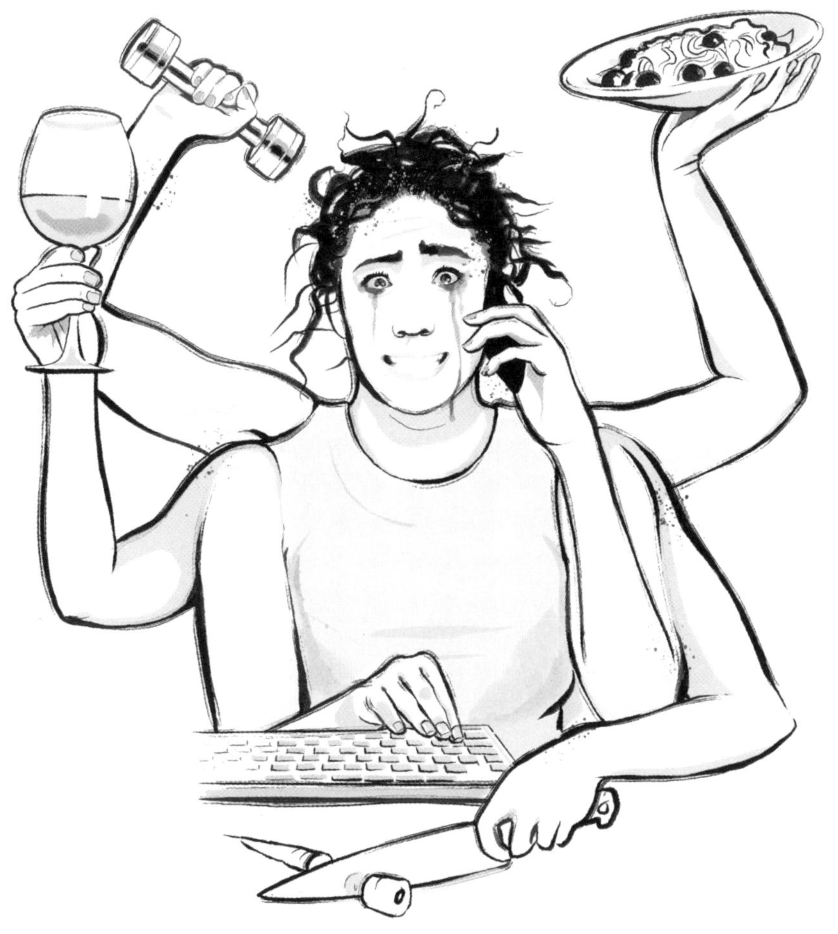

HOW REFRAMING YOUR THINKING CAN HELP

While the best results of CBT come from working with a therapist one-to-one, here are a few common thought patterns that you might experience during menopause, along with some simple ways to reframe those thoughts to reduce their power over you. If any of them sound a bit familiar, try and use the ideas opposite to change your narrative:

MIND-READING

You think: This hot flush is awful; everyone must be staring at me.

Try thinking: Everyone is far more concerned with themselves, so they won't have noticed.

'SHOULD' STATEMENTS

You think: This is a natural process; I should be able to cope better with it.

Try thinking: The menopause can be a difficult process and as such, I am coping.

CATASTROPHISING

You think: There must be something deeply wrong for me to be so forgetful.

Try thinking: Forgetfulness is a common symptom of the menopause and it doesn't mean there's a higher chance of dementia or other neurocognitive conditions.

DISCOUNTING THE POSITIVES

You think: There's nothing good about midlife; it's all downhill from here.

Try thinking: There are many positive things about this half of my life, and I will make a concerted effort to focus on them.

OVERGENERALISATION & PERFECTIONIST THINKING

You think: I made a mistake at work when I was having a bad day and I just don't think I'm good at it anymore.

Try thinking: There were countless days that I was good at my job which means I am good at it – no one's perfect after all.

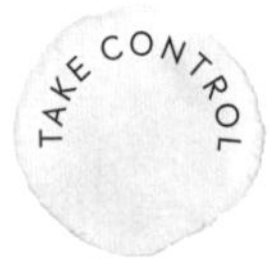

The alignment process

WITH DAWN BRESLIN, AUTHOR AND FOUNDER OF *THE HARMONIZING ACADEMY*

When my menopause hit, a choice faced me: Refuse to accept the menopause and continue to struggle upstream to try and get back to pre-menopausal me. Or start a new stage in my life, where I would cast off that which no longer suited me and use that space to focus on what I really wanted. I chose the latter, and used a technique I, and many women who have come to me for support, have found useful. It is called ***The Harmonizing Alignment Process*** *and it works via four key pillars:*

Pillar 1: Find what makes you happy

For most of us, our passion has always been there, bubbling somewhere beneath the surface of our responsibilities. MenoPAUSE is the ideal opportunity to start refocusing your lens.

Childhood photos and photos from times in our lives when we felt really happy can help here: if you have some you may want to get them out and spend time looking at them.

Try and reconnect with the happy and spontaneous you. What did you like? Running through the woods? Art? Live music? Dancing? If you take the time you can begin to hear those desires and joys whispering, telling you they are still there, begging you to reclaim your sparkle.

Forget the opinions of others and take time to list the things that energise and exhilarate you. The things that make you feel alive.

Pillar 2: Create boundaries

This is probably the toughest part. Strong boundaries are needed to ensure you free the time and energy to do what you identified in Pillar 1. Most women of menopausal age simply have too much going on to fit anything more in until they drop something. Maybe you have become an unpaid babysitter to your grandchildren five days a week and are starting to feel a bit resentful or you are the one at work everyone depends on to put in the long hours. Maybe you have some friends that drain you, but guilt makes you continue to spend time with them. You need to set boundaries to stop this and put yourself first.

Establishing strong boundaries can be hard if you are not used to it. One positive thing about that short fuse that often bubbles to the surface during menopause is that it can often give you the energy to get those boundaries in place. Difficult decisions abound in this pillar – what exactly do you need to drop to allow yourself space to flourish? Then how are you going to take steps to action them? The next pillar can help with this.

Pillar 3: Self-care

When I talk about self-care, I am not talking about a bubble bath and a magazine. I am talking about FIERCE self-care. It's giving yourself permission to really take care of yourself. To refuel your tank. And that doesn't need to be an expensive day at a spa. It might be taking a holiday alone, whether somewhere local, booking into a cheap B&B, or somewhere amazing you have always wanted to go. Or spending a day in bed with your favourite books or boxset when you are tired rather than powering on.

Often, when I talk to women and ask what they really want, they say, 'I just want to spend a few days in bed sleeping but I can't.' And sometimes they really can't, but often, with some boundary setting, it is possible. One woman got her husband to take the children to his mum's for the weekend. She then climbed into bed and stayed there for 48 hours. A pitstop, if you like, recalibrating her life. And most importantly – don't feel guilty about it. This kind of self-care is essential to give you the energy to make the changes you need.

Pillar 4: Courage

Rewriting the script of your life takes guts. Redesigning your life based on your deep desires may mean rebelling against what others expect from you. Don't expect everyone to like it!

So, it's your choice. You can fade away or have a long, hard look at your life and ruthlessly prune what no longer serves you and start planting the garden your heart desires. Accept that it might be tough – but it can also be worth it as you march to the next phase of your life with pride, strength and determination.'

CBD oil explained

CBD (short for cannabidiol) oil acts on receptors in the brain that control functions like sleep and pain. It also seems to alter blood flow in the brain. This combination of effects has been shown to help many problems that you can experience in menopause including anxiety.

As you might have guessed by the first part of that word, CBD is extracted from plants in the cannabis sativa family; these include hemp and marijuana. Don't panic, though! CBD is not going to get you high. The substance in cannabis that does that is called THC (or tetrahydrocannabinol, if you like long words). It's only found in large quantities in marijuana, and most products sold without a prescription in the UK come from hemp which naturally has very low THC levels. To further ensure this is the case, CBD products in the UK can only contain less than 0.2 per cent of THC - and most products you buy have far, far less.

HOW MUCH TO TAKE?

This is very, very hard to answer as it varies from person to person, but a starting dose of 20mg is often suggested. Try that for a few days, and if you don't get relief, increase by 20mg. Keep going until you find the dose that works for you (obviously never exceeding the maximum intake per day listed on your product). Reduce your dosage if symptoms seem to get worse again.

CBD oil labelling can be very confusing so it's best to start with a product that clearly states how many mg of CBD it contains per sweet or drop, rather than just saying what percentage of CBD is in the bottle.

IS CBD SAFE?

Research is still ongoing about all of the effects of CBD, but generally it seems that, yes, it is safe - however, you must speak to your doctor before using it if you are on any kind of medication as it can interfere with the metabolism of some drugs.

'It is commonly believed that we automatically lose our sexual desire and ability as we get older. This is absolutely not true! But certain changes do take place, and it's worth being aware of these.'

PAMELA STEPHENSON-CONNOLLY,
SEX LIFE

FOUR

Let's talk about Sex...

My Story

When I was younger, my sex drive was through the roof and climaxing was so easy. I was adventurous in the bedroom and enjoyed satisfying my voracious sexual appetite. But as soon as menopause started, I didn't even want to share a bed with my partner, let alone have sex with him. I struggled to orgasm; it took so long I just couldn't be bothered. Spending entire days in bed were no longer due to passion, but exhaustion and a desire to watch Netflix from under the duvet. It was odd to no longer feel anything when I saw someone attractive. It was like the most intimate part of me, the key to my sexuality, was letting me down. My lack of sex drive was having a destructive effect on my relationship. I felt very isolated and alone, and my partner felt rejected.

Loss of libido is common at this stage in life, and it isn't surprising. Changing hormones affect desire and sex can also become uncomfortable. Vulval skin gets thinner and can even start to rip. The clitoral hood can start to shrink back and if you have had children then the resulting scars can get thinner and older episiotomy scars can start to hurt. A menopausal vagina is very different from a young woman's vagina!

So, should we just give up? I think not. Some people are horrified about how much I talk about masturbation, lube and sex. I even see some women wince when I mention the word vagina! I have an open attitude to sex. I feel no embarrassment writing or talking about it. It is completely natural, and I just don't see what the big deal is; lube and toys are even available on the high street now.

I also regularly masturbate. I was shocked to find many women of my age never have. I recommend 3–4 times a week; it helps with vaginal dryness as it is a great way to lubricate the vagina. I find the more I 'flick my bean', the easier it is for me to climax. I've done it in the shower and once even on a sunbed! Clitoral stimulation is key for orgasm for most women – I find my bullet vibrator great for this. Do what works for you. It might take a few times, but relax and go at your own pace. As well as sexual satisfaction and faster climaxing, it is also a chance to get comfortable with your body and take control of your sexuality. When you climax, every cell in you is woken up, you glow and simply feel better.

Women experience a drop in testosterone in menopause, which is linked to a decrease in sex drive, and there is a gel available, but at the moment it is mostly used by men. I was prescribed some by a private doctor and I found it did make a difference to me personally – one to watch.

I also had to start making more of an effort. Sitting around in pyjamas with my hair scraped back was my default for months. Putting on makeup and a little spray of perfume was a huge effort some days, but when I did, I felt more like a sexual being than a sloth.

If penetration really hurts, then remember sex isn't just about penetration. Experiment with your partner and find other things that turn you both on. 'Missionary and vanilla' was how one woman I met described her sex life until the menopause. Then, after 18 months of no sex she tried experimentation that did not involve penetration. Now at 56, her sex life has never been better. Some people like to light the candles and get some music on. Others like a drink to relax them. Others fantasise and perhaps use porn. There are no rules, and it can be fun trying new things. Penetration can be helped with dilators and lubricant (I prefer silicon dilators as they are softer). I have my own lube, which is vegan and is presented in pretty packaging so I have no problem with it sitting on my bedside cabinet - even with a houseful of teenagers.

I thought I would never fancy anyone again, then one day I saw a rather muscular builder who was working, naked from the waist up. It was nice to feel a little spark. And, while I am not swinging from the chandeliers, I can say that with a bit of work and a bit of effort, there is most definitely light at the end of the tunnel.

***Don't forget:** You can still get pregnant until you have gone two years without a period if you are under 50, or a year when over 50! Meno-babies are more common than you think, so take precautions unless you fancy the patter of tiny feet. Ask your doctor which is the best contraception for you - and always use condoms with a new partner.*

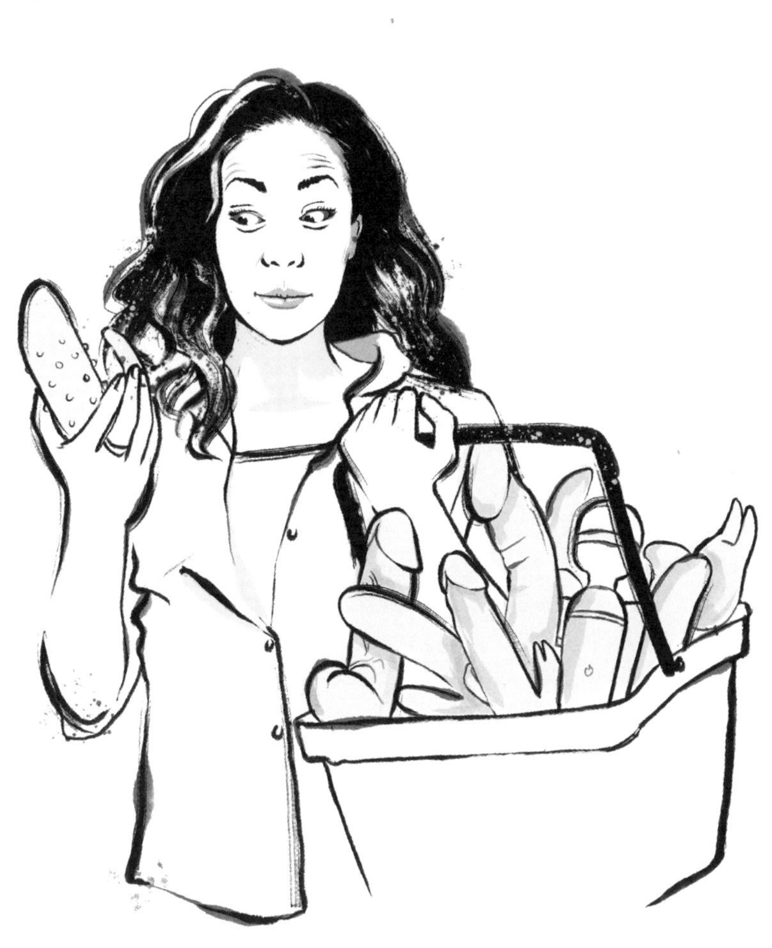

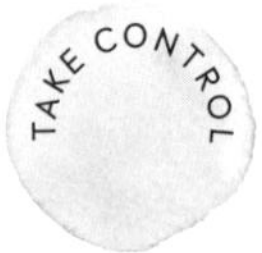

Buying Lube

My lube transformed my life. A few drops warmed on your fingers and then put around the clitoris, vulva and inside the vagina can reduce friction and make sex so much more pleasurable. But it's important to choose the right type for you, and you may need a different type than you might have tried in the past as the vaginal tissues become more sensitive post-menopause. There are different types of lube out there so here's how to choose the right one for you:

Water-based

Particularly good for menopausal women as they are kind to sensitive skin. They can be used with condoms and won't damage any sex toys. They also don't stain your sheets. They may need to be reapplied though as they are quickly absorbed by the skin.

Silicone-Based

Their silky feel makes them lovely to use and silicone is hypoallergenic so they are unlikely to irritate. They last longer than water-based lubes. They can stain sheets though and shouldn't be used with any sex toy. Hybrid lubes combine both silicone and water – check the label if you want to use these with any sex toy to make sure they are suitable.

Oil-Based

Their main benefit is they last a long time, but they can damage condoms so avoid if you are using these. They may also stain sheets or lingerie. Because they can be harder to wash away, they may linger longer, which can alter the vaginal balance – try to use them externally rather than inside the vagina.

Natural

Made with organic or vegan ingredients these don't contain chemicals called parabens that many people try to avoid as there's a belief they may be harmful to health. They can have a shorter shelf life than other lubes.

What to avoid

Lubricants that contain glycerine or any 'warming' ingredients, particularly if you suffer from vaginal dryness, as they can irritate.

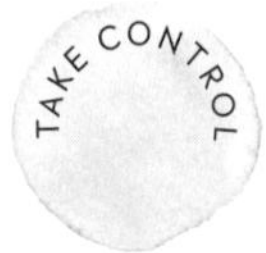

5 things to know about vibrators

They are no longer just big lumps of plastic shaped like a penis – things have changed a lot.

1. **There's not one type.** You can buy G-spot stimulators, clitoral stimulators, dildos that go inside you and suctiony-type vibes that feel a bit like a tongue. Think about what you love most during sex and try and find the vibe that simulates those feelings. Websites like **Love Honey** are really female-friendly and help explain exactly what their vibes do, or go into a store like Ann Summers or Harmony where you can see and feel how the vibes work.

2. **Try it on the end of your nose.** That's how vibrators are tested in the laboratory – the nose contains a similar amount of nerve endings to the clitoris. If you like how it feels on your nose, you might also like how it feels down below.

3. **If, maybe, you tried a vibe back in the early 80s, and didn't get on with it, try again.** Vibrator technology and design has come a long way, and many women are now involved with designing vibrators, meaning they are much more likely to hit the spot. Good female-focused companies include Dame, We Vibe and Jimmy Jane.

4. **Noise matters.** You need to be relaxed to climax and that's less likely if you think the kids can hear what's going on. Pick products that say they are quiet.

5. **You don't need to leave your partner out of all of this.** They can use the vibe on you before penetration, or devices like the We Melt are designed to sit between the two of you during intercourse.

expert view

LET'S TALK ABOUT . . . SEX IN THE MENOPAUSE

WITH CLARE PRENDERGAST, PSYCHOSEXUAL THERAPIST

The menopause is not called 'the change' for nothing. It is exactly that, a change in hormones, a change in your body, a change in the way you feel and relate to the world and your loved ones, and desire and libido can be affected by this.

Feeling sexual is strongly linked to your emotions. It's not uncommon during menopause to think you're losing your mind as the person you've got used to being isn't there anymore; that can be terrifying – and fear ain't horny! Nor are the feelings of loss that menopause can create. The obvious trigger is the disappearance of periods and fertility, but you might also feel a loss of your looks or health and that can also sap your confidence sexually. There are, however, solutions to all of these. When I work with clients who are medically focused, I refer them to a GP or gynaecologist to talk about hormone replacement therapy. Others are more interested in holistic interventions like diet, exercise, meditation supplements or body work (e.g, acupuncture, shiatsu, reflexology). There are many ways to navigate this life stage so find support that suits you.

Patience helps and doesn't come easily to everyone. Menopause can take a while, sometimes 10 years or more, and new challenges will keep coming, so be prepared for this and be willing to tweak your interventions as you move through it. Talk with your partner; it's very tempting to shut them out and believe they don't understand, particularly if they keep 'getting it wrong', but persevere. Find out how it is for them too - and try to be kind; partners tell me they are often fearful about getting things wrong and making things worse, but risk letting them learn alongside you and your sex life can be positively transformed by menopause.

If you're in a long-term relationship, what the two of you have done before probably won't be the same thing that works now. You are going to need to try new things. That might be mean bringing in lubes or vibrators and the key is to keep experimenting - don't try one lube and think, 'that smelt disgusting, I don't want to use lubes', try another. Shake things up a bit - try new locations, contexts and timings. Explore new sensations; this can be a wonderful time for new discoveries.

Also, spend time with yourself and your body; it's very easy to be self-critical now, whether it's weight gain, or whatever, and we can be really mean to ourselves during menopause. So, there's a requirement, I think, to love yourself and let your body know that you're on its side. Orgasms can become more elusive so try and move from outcome-oriented sexual activity (coming) to process-oriented sexual activity (exploring what feels good) both with your partner and alone. More self-awareness can also help you communicate with your partner about what you want from them when they are touching your body. It's not their sole responsibility to get it right, so keep talking.

Finally, it's worth noting that quite often desire will kick in if you just get started. So, even if you are not in the mood, often, if you instead think, 'oh, go on let's just give it a whirl', you might find yourself having quite a nice time.

“

‘My sex life actually got better after the menopause – I was no longer worried about getting pregnant and we became a bit more adventurous after I got the confidence to ask for what I really wanted in bed.’

'Hey, this isn't an old lady disease! We aren't old! We are strong and dammit, we are beautiful and sexy too.'

LISA JEY DAVIS – *GETTING OVER YOUR OVARIES: HOW TO MAKE THE 'CHANGE OF LIFE' YOUR BITCH*

FIVE

Vagina SOS

My Story

Ladies, we need to talk about our vaginas. We spend thousands of pounds on the skin on our face but only one in three of us seek help for what happens to the skin of the vagina during menopause. See, just as the fall in oestrogen affects the skin on the face, it does the same to the skin and tissues of the vulva and vagina, which can get dry and itchy. The walls thin and the vagina loses its moisture and softness. Not only can this make things generally uncomfortable, it can also make sex sore. If you then stop having sex because of that, things get worse even faster.

A young vaginal area is naturally plump and wet, but as we age that changes. In fact, the girls at my waxing place once told me that they can spot a menopausal vagina, or one that's not being used, a mile away. 'It's just not as plump,' they said. I asked my gynaecologist if this was true and she said yes, you can absolutely tell.

I had noticed mine was getting a bit redder than normal. When I had my coil taken out, the nurse said it looked like I had the beginning of vaginal atrophy. I had no idea what she was talking about. She explained that I was experiencing thinning, drying and inflammation of the walls of the vagina. I just sighed, thinking, 'What else is the menopause going to throw at me?' I had assumed I had thrush and was using thrush medication to try and relieve it. No wonder it didn't work. I then looked further into it and was shocked at just how bad it could get. Women with vaginal atrophy have a greater chance of chronic infections and for some it can get to the point they can't even wear jeans and even riding a bike feels like sitting on a bonfire. Some of the photographs of just how bad it can get are on the internet and really shocked me.

Whether you are experiencing symptoms or not, you should be familiar with what's going on down there. This isn't something we normally do – when I mentioned to one group of ladies that all women should regularly look and check their vulvas, I was met with horror – one woman exclaimed, 'There is no way I am going to look down there – no way.' Why the bloody hell not? We are regularly reminded to check our breasts and get advice if there are any noticeable changes, so why not the same with our vulvas? I regularly look at mine with a mirror and, yes it does feel a bit odd to begin with, but you quickly become aware of what is normal for you and can pick up on any changes. With five types of gynaecological cancers out there, knowing what is and isn't normal for you can literally mean the difference between life and death. If you do notice something, go to the doctor and insist they look.

Another 'gift' from the menopause can be incontinence; anything from an occasional 'peeze' (where you leak a little bit of urine when you sneeze or laugh) to full on flooding. Incontinence pad adverts frustrate me about this. They suggest it is normal to wee yourself and you should just stick a pad in, but it's important to tackle this. Vaginal atrophy and/or a condition called lichen sclerosis (a skin condition causing itchy white patches on the genitals) combined with a urine-soaked pad can essentially lead to nappy rash – and no one needs that at 50.

So, what did I do? Well, I am a woman of extremes, so I decided to have vaginal rejuvenation. For me, this worked, but it isn't for everyone. It involved three sessions over three months of laser treatment then a 'top-up' session every year. This puts the collagen back in and plumps everything back up. Twice a week I also use an oestrogen suppository as the pelvic floor is very oestrogen receptive – as my next expert explains...

expert view

LET'S TALK ABOUT . . . VAGINAL DRYNESS

WITH JANE LEWIS, CAMPAIGNER

Vaginal dryness, also known as vaginal atrophy or genitourinary syndrome of menopause, can affect many women around menopause. Dryness makes it sound like a slight inconvenience, atrophy like it's all shrivelling up, and a 'syndrome' amongst other things, implies it's in the head, which it most definitely is not – the problem is between our legs.

The vagina, vulva, bladder and the pelvic floor all love oestrogen so when it declines it can, and does, have serious repercussions for many women. The lack of oestrogen basically makes the vagina and surrounding area weaker, thinner and easily irritated. The bladder becomes more prone to urine infections because bacteria can take hold much easier.

The thinning of the vagina means sex can be painful, and at worst, impossible, while the vulva

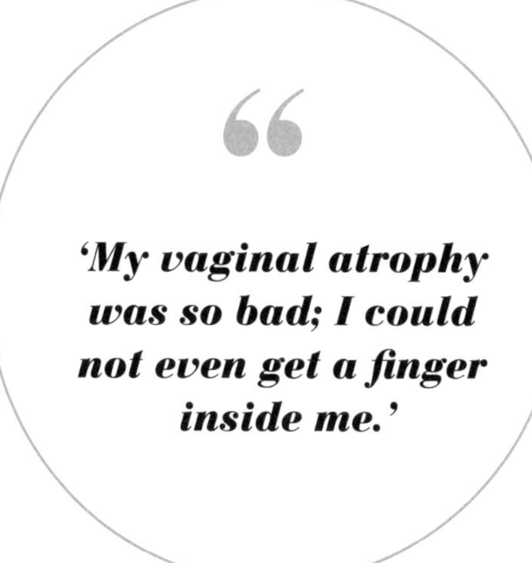

skin can become so thin that a simple smear test, which was once easy, becomes painful or impossible. The skin can become red, itch and feel sore all the time with a burning feeling that makes wearing pants or even sitting down uncomfortable or impossible for some – and as for riding a horse… well, forget that!

Sounds horrid, doesn't it, and almost made up? Well, no, this is me, and potentially over 70 per cent of women in some form or another. My issues started at 45 when I was still having periods and considered perimenopausal – it's another huge myth that these symptoms only happen post-menopause.

If this happens to you, don't ignore the symptoms. With proper care and support life can be made so much more comfortable!

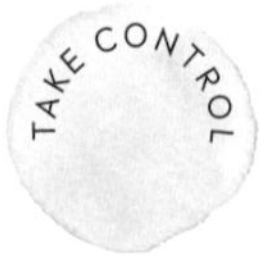

Pussy power

If you are experiencing vaginal dryness and discomfort, don't panic! There is plenty that you can do to help make life more comfortable:

1. **Start by communicating**
Dryness can be a very difficult subject to broach, even with your doctor, let alone your partner, but communication is key to understanding and finding a way forward.

2. **Take your time during sex**
Many women first notice the symptoms of vaginal dryness during sex, because the vagina during menopause, may shrink a little and expand less easily. The more aroused you become, the more the vagina expands, so explain to your partner that you might need a little bit extra help getting turned on and wet – but that you'll enjoy everything a lot more if you both take the time.

3. **Ask your doctor about specific oestrogen cream and other solutions**

This is applied to the vagina a couple of times a week and restores oestrogen levels in the area. After just a couple of weeks of using it, your vagina will plump up and you'll find it easier to get wet. This can be used by most women, including many who have had breast cancer and can't use HRT in other forms. You can also deliver oestrogen direct to the vagina via pessaries, tablets or a vaginal ring, which stays in place for three months at a time.

4. **Get familiar with your vulva and vagina**

If you have never looked between your legs, get a mirror and give it a go. Check it's all roughly the same colour – there shouldn't be areas of much paler or darker skin. Look for new lumps and bumps or sore spots. If anything doesn't seem right, then get checked out by a doctor.

5. **Know your lingo**

It will be easier to explain what's happening if you understand your genital anatomy. The area outside your body is your vulva – this consists of the vaginal lips, of which there are two sets, and the clitoris. The area that goes up inside you is the vagina.

MAKING SMEARS MORE COMFORTABLE

Everyone thinks when I start talking about masturbation it's just Meg Mathews, rock chick, banging on about sex again, but when I lost my libido I felt I was dead from the waist down and that didn't just mean in the bedroom. It also meant I didn't want to go for my smear test. I was just 'nah, don't need to bother, nothing is going on down there, I'm not thinking about it anymore. I'll just cuddle up with my dogs, watch my Netflix box sets and forget about it.'

But, you need smears until you're 64 for a reason. About a third of the cases of cervical cancer that are diagnosed each year happen in women over 50, and regular smears will catch things early, making treatment far more likely to be successful. And remember, after 50 you only need to go every five years. SO, you can do a few things to make the process a bit more comfortable.

SPEAK TO YOUR DOCTOR BEFORE YOU GO

Vaginal oestrogen cream helps plump up the walls of the vagina and makes the test more comfortable. Even if you don't want to use it all the time, you can just use it for a few weeks prior to a smear appointment and it will make things easier.

DON'T USE LUBRICANT

It might seem like a good idea to use lubricant, but don't as it can affect the sample, which increases the chance of you having to go back for a second try. Your doctor will use a gel that won't interfere. That goes for about 24 hours before the test too.

SHIFT POSITION IF ITS NOT GOING WELL

A smear test collects a sample of cells from the neck of the cervix, but as we get older, the area where these cells are found actually moves higher up into the vagina. If you're having problems, ask the practitioner if taking the smear in a different position might help. The test can be done on your side, or with your hips resting on something – I even had one friend where the doctor put their bum on a telephone book to get them in the right position.

WEAR A SKIRT

You can pull it up easily and you'll feel a bit less exposed as they take the sample – the more you relax, the easier it is. If you're not having sex at the moment, it can suddenly become more embarrassing to let someone poke about down there, so anything that relaxes you will help.

ASK FOR A THIN SPECULUM

I had no idea these come in different shapes and sizes until recently but they do, and a narrower, flatter type of speculum is often more comfortable for the more mature vagina.

DON'T PANIC IF YOU GET CALLED BACK

Chances are it's not because there's something wrong. The cells of the cervix don't detach as easily as we get older and this can mean even the best smear test taker won't always get a good sample, so you might have to come back for them to have another go.

expert view

LET'S TALK ABOUT . . . YOUR PELVIC FLOOR

WITH ELAINE MILLER, PELVIC PHYSIOTHERAPIST

Women often find it awkward or embarrassing to talk about pelvic floor, leaking pee, etc (unless you are one of Meg's friends, in which case, I suspect talking about sex and genitals is compulsory), but healthcare professionals have seen and heard it all before so please come and see us! We get a real kick out of women becoming free of worry and living their life without thinking about their bladder and bowel.

Some women who come into my clinic weep because of what they are going through; incontinence and sexual dysfunction can be devastating to a woman's life. Feelings of being alone and anxiety that nothing can be done are also common – but I can tell you both are untrue. Although fairly common, pelvic floor issues are never 'normal' or to be put up with, and there is so much that you can do to improve the situation.

Many women don't leak pee (or poo) until they are menopausal, which can be a shock. It happens because loss of oestrogen affects all your soft tissues, including the ligaments in your pelvis that some of the pelvic floor muscles attach to. That affects their ability to support your bladder, so you might start to leak when you sneeze or cough.

Understanding what your pelvic floor is and what it does can help. The muscles are arranged like a hammock in your pelvis and support your bladder, uterus, vagina and rectum. They aren't fixed like a floor but move up and down in time with your breath. They should be strong and reactive enough to contract to keep the neck of your bladder closed when you laugh, cough and sneeze and to resist impact forces when you run, dance or jump, and be able to help you 'hold on' if there is no toilet available.

Leakages etc, affect around one in three women, so you're definitely not alone. Pelvic floor exercises (see page 91) are a great place to start, so even if you aren't experiencing any leaking yet, make sure you do them often! The stats show that pelvic floor exercises help about 70 per cent of women with incontinence issues, and for the rest, more specialist pelvic physiotherapy is known to be effective. Options like medication, pessaries and surgery can also be considered. Regular pelvic floor exercises can help to manage prolapse (around 50 per cent of women aged over 50 have a prolapse of some degree, whether they've had children or not)

Like any other muscle, your pelvic floor muscles also have to be able to relax – a tight, inflexible pelvic floor can cause as many problems as a weak one, and exercises help this too. I know it is really hard to remember to do them! I think we could use sex to 'sell' pelvic floor exercises, as your pelvic floor has an important role in your sexual function. An orgasm is, in part, a flickering contraction of the muscles, so if your pelvic floor is strong and responsive, then so are your orgasms. How's that for an incentive?

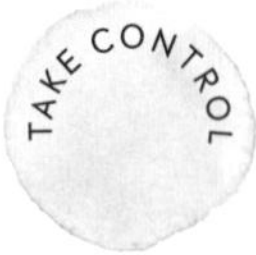

How to strengthen your pelvic floor

The pelvic floor is a muscle, and like any muscle it needs exercise to keep it healthy. Over to Elaine to explain how to work it:

There are two types of pelvic floor contraction: a long hold and quick flicks. The long hold will help you strengthen your muscles especially for those times when you need to hold on, the second will stop leaking if you laugh or jump.

Long hold exercises:

1. Take a deep breath in, sigh out as you squeeze and lift your bumhole.

2. Hold for a count of 10 (keep breathing) and relax. Don't worry if you can't hold it for a count of 10, keep practising, and as you get stronger, you'll be able to hold on for longer.

Quick flicks exercises:

1. This time, quickly tense then release the muscles, 10 times. Try not to hold your breath as you do this.

If you are experiencing leakages, do both those exercises three times a day, for three months. Once you are dry do the exercises once a day, every day, for maintenance.

If, after three months of doing exercises, you are still not dry or if you get pain when you do the exercises, are not sure what you are doing, or they just don't work, then go to see a specialist pelvic health physiotherapist. We work directly on training the muscles in this area, just like a sports physiotherapist might help strengthen your back or legs after injury. To find one, search online for 'pelvic health' or 'women's health' physiotherapy.

Some health services have a self-referral system, some need GP referral, and some physios work privately, so ask at the clinic what you need to do to make an appointment.

While you're working on the exercises, pads are a useful tool to protect from leaks. Although remember that while a pad can help confidence, it won't fix anything. Do your pelvic floor exercises, don't put up with leaking!

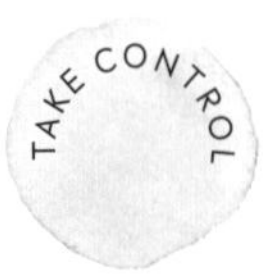

Reducing the risk of UTIs

Urinary tract infections (UTIs) occur when bacteria like E. coli that normally live harmlessly in the back passage of the bowel, enter the urinary tract where they don't belong, and start to multiply. At any age, women are far more prone to UTIs than men because our urethra (the tube you urinate from) is closer to the back passage, meaning bacteria can more easily infiltrate it. At menopause, the risks increase further because falling oestrogen levels affect the levels of protective bacteria in the urethra; as levels of these fall it increases the chance that other bacteria might take hold. Trying to reduce your risk of UTIs is mostly about you working on reducing the amount of bacteria that might enter the system. Here's how to do it:

- **Always wipe front to back** (not the other way round) when you go to the toilet.
- **Use the toilet after sex.** Sex can push bacteria closer to the urethra but urinating afterwards flushes it out.
- **Don't wear thong underwear.** This fits closer to the genitals than other styles and can help move bacteria from the back passage to the urethra.
- **Consider taking a supplement called d-mannose.** It's a sugar that seems to stop E. coli bacteria sticking to the walls of the urinary tract – making it easier for you to pass them out.

Even though UTIs might become more common during menopause, you should still take them seriously. See your GP if you notice blood in your urine or if your symptoms don't improve after 2-3 days. Ask for an urgent appointment if you have pain in your sides or lower back, develop a temperature or get an upset stomach/vomiting – this can be a sign that the infection has reached the kidneys and this should always be taken seriously.

'When my sleep began to go awry in my late 40s, I put it down to working too hard, juggling life etc. It was only while researching my book, The Good Menopause Guide, *that the penny finally dropped.'*

LIZ EARLE, AUTHOR AND WELLNESS EXPERT

SIX

Wake me up when it's all over

My Story

Sleep, or more specifically, the lack of it, is a big issue for so many menopausal women. If I sleep well, then I rise knowing I can take on all the challenges the day throws at me. But if my sleep is interrupted then I spend the day tired and grumpy. I'm also likely to make poor food choices and not work out as the fatigue worsens over the day.

I had terrible problems with sleep during the menopause. After my first night sweat I honestly thought someone had poured a bucket of water all over me. I remember getting out of bed, literally dripping like I'd got out of a pool. The sheets were soaked, so I had to wake my partner, change everything and by the time I'd done all that I was wide awake!

It took a bit of time to get my sleep pattern right. I used to go to bed and watch telly while playing on my phone with the iPad charging beside me. I have now completely digitally detoxed my bedroom. No electronics at all. My bedroom is very tranquil, and I have decorated it to make it calm. I also have shungite around my bed; this is a black crystal from Russia, and it is believed to protect against waves from technology. The benefits I have read about it include detoxifying and purifying your body by absorbing negative energies and toxins (and there are a lot of them in London!). It might not be for everyone but doing this really helped me get a good night's sleep.

I also started a regular sleep pattern. I find going to bed around 10pm then waking at 5am suits me best. If I happen to go back to sleep after 5am, I tend to have awful dreams and feel a bit sick when I finally wake. Also, if I am up after 10pm I get really thrown. A couple of drops of CBD oil and some warm milk helps me nod off. I also find it helps to avoid any intense exercise after about 5pm.

These steps helped me and I sleep like a baby now. Well, except when my dog Ziggy decides to sleep with me! He's always waking me up. He's in the bed, out of the bed, under the duvet, on top of the duvet. If there's one thing that's going to mess with my sleep now, it's Ziggy.

expert view

LET'S TALK ABOUT . . . WHAT HAPPENS WITH SLEEP

WITH LIZ EARLE, AUTHOR AND WELLBEING EXPERT

When my sleep began to go awry in my late 40s, I put it down to working too hard, juggling life as a new mother (I had a late baby aged 47 which somewhat blurred my hormonal decline), coping with teenagers, ageing parents, work pressures of running a business as well as a farm and a charity.

Not once did I even consider my lowering levels of oestrogen could be to blame.

It was only while researching my book, T*he Good Menopause Guide*, that the penny finally dropped. As part of my research process I interviewed Dr Louise Newson, who you met at the start of this book, and she talked me through the 34 or so symptoms of perimenopause. It was like pieces of a jigsaw suddenly fitting together: The waking up at 4am with a racing heartbeat, the debilitating headaches that painkillers didn't touch, the irrational anxiety over small issues that shouldn't really have bothered me. Even the onset of mild tinnitus was an unrecognised symptom for me - one that I only appreciated after taking HRT for a year or so when I suddenly realised my hearing was crystal clear again.

I finally understood the fact that, as we have oestrogen receptors all over our bodies, including our brain and even our inner ears, even the slightest decline in our oestrogen levels will obviously trigger some kind of symptom, from mild through to moderate or severe - and sleep can be one of those.

On Dr Newson's advice, I saw my GP who (thankfully) immediately prescribed the body identical form of oestrogen gel (made from the wild yam plant, so a botanical that fits with my general philosophy) and a body identical micronised progesterone. I can honestly say that I had the best night's sleep in years after just one application. It was truly transformational - and my overwhelmingly positive experience is one reason why I work so hard now on telling other women how it helped me.

As an overly busy mid-life woman, still running businesses, juggling family pressures and all the usual work-life balance stuff that so many of us try to do, having my sleep restored has enabled me to continue to do the above in a better way than before. And for this I am truly thankful.

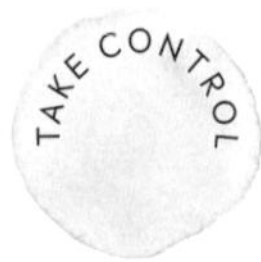

Natural tips to improve sleep

WITH CAROLINE GASKIN, HOMEOPATH AND NATURAL HEALTH PRACTITIONER

While HRT helped Liz (see page 99), if you don't want to, or can't use it, there is also a lot you can do to help with menopause-related sleep problems naturally. Some very simple ideas include taking a cool shower before bedtime, stopping screen time by 9pm (including switching off the Wi-Fi) and reducing excess light in the bedroom.

But on top of this, recent studies show that glyphosate (a type of pesticide) combined with other toxins in the environment might be affecting our glands, including the pineal gland that releases the sleep hormone melatonin. Eating organic can help reduce exposure to glyphosate and other toxins. Taking a probiotic thought to clear glyphosate from the gut may also help.

“

‘After 22 years of sleeping together in the same bed, the menopause finally made me decide to move to the spare room.’

I use a product in practice containing a strain called *Bacillus coagulans* (among others) which may help.

Natural sources of melatonin (the sleep hormone) can also help – tart cherry juice is one of these and having a glass before bedtime can make dropping off to sleep easier. Some women also do well on a combination of homeopathic sleep remedies such as *valaeriana*, *passiflora* and *coffea* and I often add a homeopathic version of melatonin to the mix.

Lastly, cleansing and supporting the liver is fundamental for reducing insomnia, hot flushes, night sweats, breast health and headaches. You’ll find a few more tips on this on page 152.

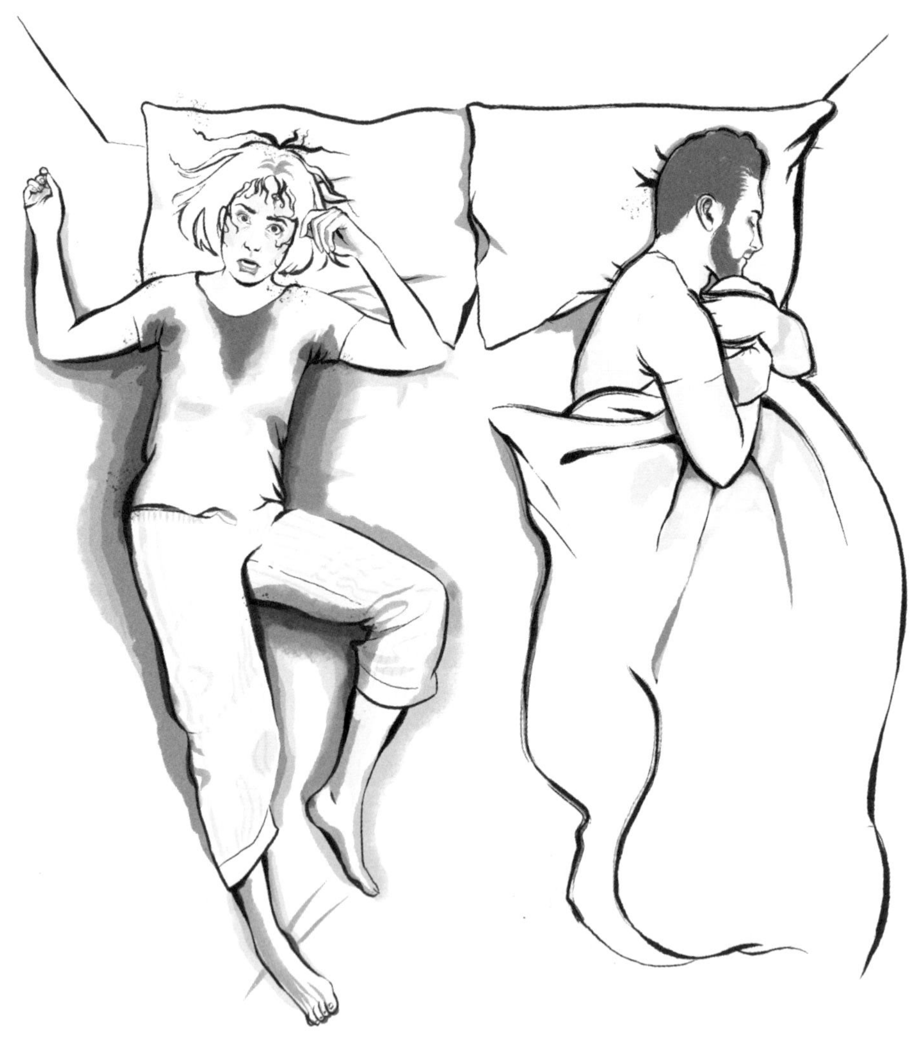

Give your bedroom a menopause makeover

Night sweats are likely to happen during menopause and while getting your bedroom in shape won't stop them, it may make them less uncomfortable. Here are some things to try:

- **Swap to cotton bedding:** Cotton sheets and pillow covers help wick away sweat, which keeps you cooler. But don't get too high a thread count. A recent study conducted by bedding company Casper found the higher the thread count the worse people said they slept. One possible reason is that the high thread count sheets trap air and humidity which will just make you hotter. Pick sheets with a 400 thread count.

- **Swap to natural nightwear:** Cotton or linen nightwear helps keep you cooler as the skin can breathe more easily. Also look for mixed blends containing bamboo, which is a great natural wicking fabric. Brands like Esteem, Cool Jams and Nite Sweatz are particularly designed to combat night sweats.

- **Sort out the room temperature:** The best temperature for sleep is 18-20°C. If your bedroom is much warmer than that, try and lower the temperature with a fan or open a window if it's safe.

- **Never look at the clock:** If you start to worry about losing sleep, it can create a state of arousal that makes it much harder to drop back off, so don't look at your phone, watch or alarm clock if you wake up. If you have a clock radio, turn it to face the wall so you can't see what the time is.

HOW TO PEP YOURSELF UP AFTER A BAD NIGHT

If you do have a bad night, you're going to feel a bit weary the next day, but there are a few tips and tricks that can help maximise and make the most of the energy you do have:

GET SOME NATURAL LIGHT

Open the curtains/blinds and get some natural light into your bedroom. This switches off the production of sleep hormones and starts the energising process.

HIT THE SHOWER

Use a citrus- or mint-scented shower gel as these scents can help pep up your brain and revive you.

TELL YOURSELF YOU ACTUALLY GOT ENOUGH SLEEP

I know that might sound stupid, but studies have shown that if you tell yourself you feel fine after a bit of a rough night, you actually perform better than if you worry about it.

COFFEE CAN HELP BUT, DON'T GO GRANDE

Researchers from Harvard Medical School suggest that if you're drinking it to wake you up, you're better to drink three to four quarter cups of coffee throughout the day than one large one first thing. If you are thirsty, drink water.

'PULSE' YOUR WORK

If you're tired, you might find it a bit harder to focus for long periods, so work in short bursts. There's a technique called Pomodoro that has you setting an alarm for 25 minutes. For that time you work on your task solely and totally. At the end of the 25 minutes, take a recharge break for 3–5 minutes. Then do another 25 minutes.

EAT A LOW-CARB LUNCH

While it might seem like a good idea to load up on energy-giving carbohydrates to get you through the day, it can increase your need for an afternoon nap. Have a small portion of wholegrain carbohydrates accompanied by some protein and vegetables, which creates more balanced blood sugar levels.

‘Some women talk about it happening overnight but it crept up on me.’

RUTH LANGSFORD, TV PRESENTER

SEVEN

Look alive: Skin-saving beauty and style tips

My Story

My skin changed so much when I hit menopause. The hormones that repaired and plumped my skin started to decrease. My face became so much drier and more sensitive. Wrinkles deepened and my skin got thinner and more prone to redness. I also started to get quite itchy skin. On top of the hormonal-based changes, the past started to catch up with me too and my former excessive alcohol intake and exposure to the sun both started to take their toll. I grew up in South Africa and didn't really bother with sunscreen - and I can now see the damage that caused.

No longer could I just nick my daughter's face masks and beauty treatments; I had to really think about what I was putting on my skin and be so much gentler with it. I am also now adamant that anything I use must be vegan and organic with recyclable packaging. I still love the sun but make sure my moisturiser has a high SPF to prevent further sun damage. I use my own MegsMenopause product, S.W.A.L.K Hyaluronic Acid Serum with my moisturiser as it adds extra hydration. I am also obsessed with Face Gym which is a full workout for the face. I go weekly to a local salon for a session. I can't lie though - I do have a bit of other help. I have Botox regularly and I have also had laser resurfacing. I haven't had any other surgery but am not ruling it out - I am looking at a neck lift and maybe getting my eyes done.

I don't just stop at my face though. I continue skincare down to my neck, chest and the rest of my body, plus, I body brush. This involves brushing the body with a natural brush in long, firm strokes. It sloughs off dead skin cells, encourages drainage of the lymph nodes and increases circulation. I also enjoy baths with Epsom salts. They are expensive so I buy them in bulk then decant them into a pretty white container in the bathroom.

The good news... One thing that did improve with menopause was my hair, which got thicker, which I think was due to the HRT I was using, although it might just have been a change to a healthier lifestyle. The colour needs a bit of help now (I'm mousy brown with a liberal sprinkling of grey!!) so every 6-8 weeks I go and get it coloured. I tend to change round my hair products as I find my hair gets used to them and they don't work so well after a couple of months. My eyebrows are a bit wild (I am very glad of the current trend for big eyebrows...) and are also a bit grey so I also get them tidied and coloured regularly.

In terms of makeup, I do think less is more as you get older. My makeup bag now consists of tinted moisturiser with a high SPF, mascara and lipstick. I have a few more tips on page 112. I do get shellac nails as they make my fingers look longer, but they do wreck my real nails. I keep trying to leave my nails natural to strengthen them, but that only ever lasts a few days, then I end up getting a new set put on!

It's also important not to give up on style just because menopause has kicked in. I have always adored fashion. I remember hitchhiking to London from Norfolk to buy a pair of Vivienne Westwood shoes that I had been saving for from my pay working at a fish and chip shop. I worked in fashion and spent every penny on it – often living on beans on toast for the full month so I could buy something to make me look good. That obsession has never stopped. I still really enjoy getting dressed up rock-chick style if I am going out. During the day, though, I am mainly in casual activewear, and if I have been out all day I love coming back, having a bath and putting my pyjamas on – even if it is just 4pm! You may need to dress around the hot flushes if they're hitting, and I found layers were the key to dealing with the sweats in winter – my go-to outfit is a vest, a baggy T-shirt then a jumper, and a big cashmere wrap and gloves so that I can take things on and off when I need to. Summer it is floaty dresses and sandals.

I used to be so paranoid about how I looked. I battled with myself when I was in the public eye as the tabloids and magazines would comment on my weight. I felt short and stocky and not at all waif-like, which was the 'in' way to look. Ironically, this made me comfort eat, which of course led to gaining more weight. I'd jump from fad diet to fad diet. But something has clicked and I'm comfortable in my own skin. I accept I have short legs but appreciate they are strong, healthy legs. I look in the mirror and say affirmations and have a huge gratitude for my life, taking one day at a time. My happiness is peace and acceptance of myself.

So, now, over to one of my favourite skin experts, Dr Nigma Talib, who works magic on so many celebrities, talk about why skin changes when menopause starts – and then she will talk hair with leading trichologist Anabel Kingsley.

expert view

LET'S TALK ABOUT . . . SKIN

WITH DR NIGMA TALIB, NATUROPATHIC DOCTOR

Oestrogen is good for skin. In fact, it's possibly the most important hormone when it comes to keeping skin feeling and looking youthful, so when levels start to fall it's not surprising that changes in appearance occur.

We lose around 1 per cent in skin thickness each year after menopause and as much of 30 per cent of our collagen in the five years afterwards, leading to an increase in lines and wrinkles and a loss of firmness. Oestrogen also helps skin retain moisture more effectively, which means skin can become drier after menopause.

Falling oestrogen levels can also make the mast cells in the skin over-sensitive, leading to an increase in irritation or allergies. Lastly, the change in the balance of hormones can lead to a dominance of androgen hormones and the development of adult acne.

Hormone replacement therapy can help many of these areas – research has shown that post-menopausal women supplementing with oestrogen were less likely to develop drier skin and had fewer lines and wrinkles than those not using it, for example, but it's not the only thing you can use. It's also super important to give the skin topical support with a good skincare regime.

The perfect menopause skincare plan

- Start with exfoliation. Oestrogen affects skin cell turnover, so the rate of this falls when oestrogen does, but exfoliation can help create faster turnover and a brighter look. Faster cell renewal can also help prevent blockages and breakouts related to adult acne. Both glycolic acids or salicylic acids help here; they both dissolve the bonds that hold dead skin cells onto the surface. Glycolic acids are particularly good for those with more mature skin as they also stimulate the production of collagen and elastin, but salicylic acid can be better if you have oily skin. It's also particularly good for those with acne or skin that tends to break out as it has anti-microbial and anti-inflammatory properties.

- You should use moisturiser daily but also invest in a good serum containing hyaluronic acid to further boost hydration. Hyaluronic acid can contain up to 1000 times its own weight in water making it key to plump, youthful looking skin, but by the time we reach our mid-40s, we only make about half as much as we need so some external help is needed. If your skin is sensitive, look at products containing probiotics; these can help balance the skin's microbiome and reinforce its protective barrier. Some forms have also been shown to fight the bacteria that cause acne.

- Each night use a serum or night moisturiser, ideally one that contains plant stem cells. They are extremely beneficial to the skin as they are taken from the cells that protect plants against environmental damage. Two of the hardiest botanicals on the planet that you might spot in products are the Uttwiler Spatlauber apple (famed because it can be stored for weeks without starting to shrivel) or the Alpine rose (which grows 3200 metres above sea level and yet protects itself beautifully against the high levels of UV radiation found at that altitude).

- Plant stem cells have a strong antioxidant and anti-inflammatory effect, so used during the day they can help to protect against UV sun damage and prevent wrinkles, but at night they help skin regenerate against damage. They can also promote the production of new collagen. Products containing stem cells can be expensive so it's important to choose reputable brands that justify the cost. I like Swisscode and you'll also find plant stem cells in my serum, Dr Nigma Serum No 1.

expert view

LET'S TALK ABOUT . . . HAIR

WITH ANABEL KINGSLEY, CONSULTANT TRICHOLOGIST

As Meg points out, hair can get thicker at menopause as the right HRT can definitely benefit your hair by boosting levels of falling oestrogen. Some women also find their hair and scalp get less oily now. However, it's more common that women notice their hair getting thinner. There are two types of thinning that can occur and you can have one, or both. The first is an increase in shedding that can happen at the beginning of menopause as oestrogen falls. It's not permanent, it only last 4–6 months, but it can be quite worrying when you see a lot of hair coming out when you brush. Thickening shampoos and conditioners can help disguise hair loss until things readjust.

The second type of thinning is caused by the shift in the ratio of oestrogen to testosterone that occurs at menopause. Women who have a genetic predisposition that means their hair follicles are sensitive to testosterone can be affected by this. Testosterone shortens the hair growth cycle and can also miniaturise the hair follicles so that hair grows through thinner. This type of hair thinning is more gradual than the shedding, and rather than finding hair in your

> “
>
> ***‘I realised I’d been using the same skincare and makeup since I was 17 – it was now over three decades later. I booked some time with a department store and left with a full new set of skincare and makeup.’***

brush, you start to notice your scalp becoming more visible or your parting getting wider. If you do notice it happening, products containing a drug called minoxidil can help slow the changes. At Philip Kingsley we also sell stimulating scalp drops that contain anti-androgens which can help, but they do need a doctor’s prescription. Again, thickening shampoos can be used to disguise thinning hair but they won’t stop it happening.

MEG'S MAKEUP TIPS FOR MENOPAUSE

Wearing makeup can be difficult during the menopause as hot sweats can cause makeup to come off. I've found a few simple product swaps can help keep things in place:

- First, start with a sweat-proof or oil-free moisturiser to keep your skin healthy and hydrated through the day (note: sweat is not hydrating).
- Always use primer for both your face and eye makeup since it'll hold on to your makeup for longer. Plus, primer can fill in and smooth out wrinkles.
- If you wear foundation, stick with long-wear liquid foundation instead of powder foundation (which doesn't mix well with sweat). If hot flushes are causing redness, avoid blush.
- For eye makeup, use waterproof products, like waterproof mascara and smudge-free waterproof eyeliner, and avoid your lower lid, which tends to be the first thing to smudge down.
- Finally, opt for lipstain instead of lipstick since it'll last longer and won't smudge off with the heat.

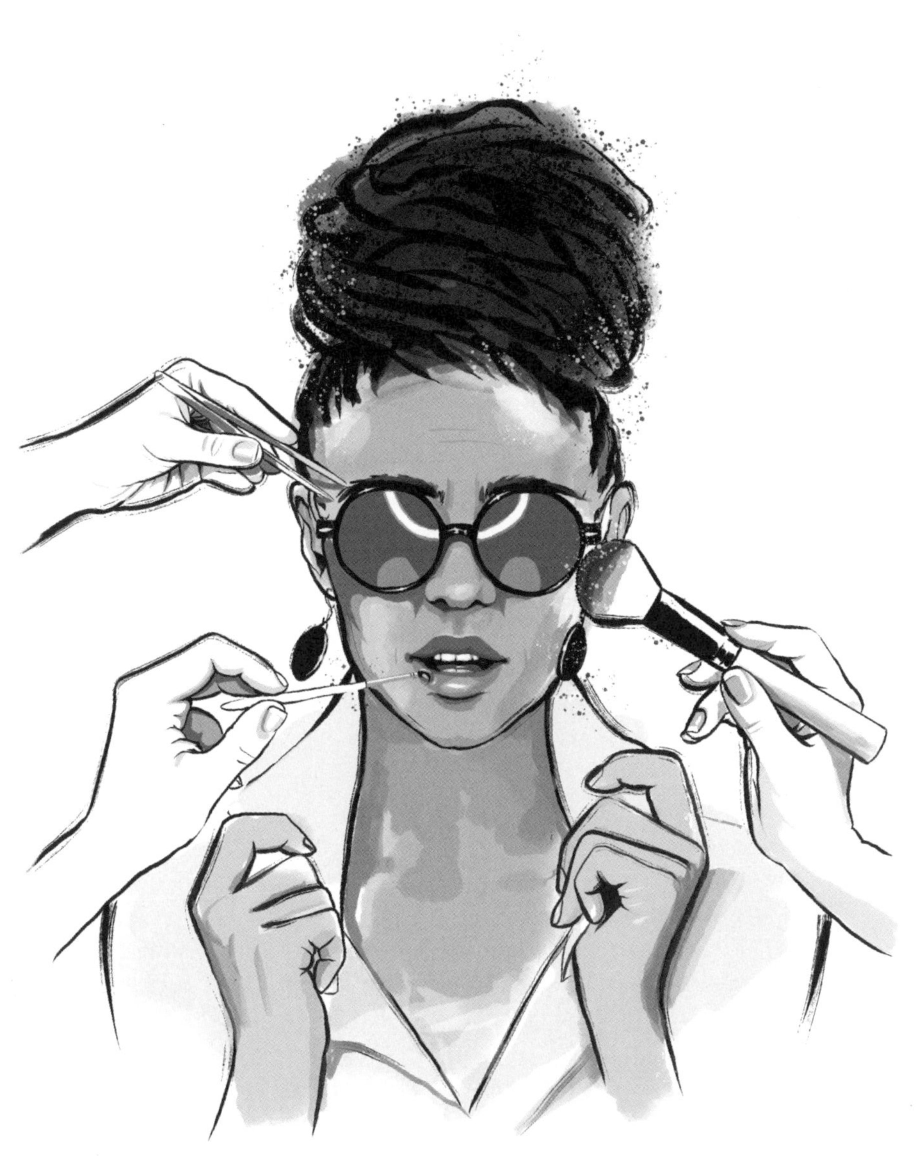

Products I like

I am lucky to be sent many complimentary products and have tried many brands over the years. I get asked a lot what I use so thought I would list some of my favourites for those who are keen to find out:

MegsMenopause S.W.A.L.K

Premium Hyaluronic Acid Serum: Hyaluronic acid stops skin being dry and this has one of the highest percentages out there – you can use it with your normal moisturiser to give it a boost.

MegsMenopause Rosey Rain

When you're feeling a bit overwhelmed or getting a flush at work, a quick spritz of this and some breathing exercises (see page 56) really calms things down.

Weleda

Another great natural brand. I really trust their products – my favourites are the lavender oil and creams.

Mio skin products

This is a vegan, organic brand that I love – they have all sorts of face and body products. I particularly like their bath range.

Aesop

I love the lip balm, hand cream, body cream – in fact, anything Aesop. I love their packaging and everything else about them.

L'Oréal Keratin

For my hair I use L'Oréal Keratin shampoo and conditioner and every few weeks I do a protein Aveda treatment at home.

Kat Burki

I'm using the Super Peptide Firming Crème and Retin-C Treatment Complex at the moment – I swap skincare a lot but I think this brand is coming out top of my list right now.

Studio10 Makeup

This is really good for more mature skin. Everything is very soft to apply and it's very hydrating. You're not trying to put on a rough brown glitter than sinks in every crevice in your eyelid like with some ranges.

Institut Esthederm Adaptasun

I like to have a year-round tan so use Institut Esthederm Adaptasun sunscreen and after sun.

Fashion and jewellery

My favourite designers include: Rixo, Ganni, Studio B, Zara, Raey and American Vintage (I love their cotton T-shirts). For workout gear, I love Unicorn, Nike and Sweaty Betty. I swear by Balenciaga trainers (comfortable and look good) and Gucci loafers. And not forgetting Missoni for bikinis! I love gold jewellery, in particular the long necklaces from Celine and my necklaces with M on them

'After one day on bioidentical oestrogen I felt the veil lift. After three days the sky was bluer, my brain was no longer fuzzy, my memory was sharper.'

OPRAH WINFREY,
TV MOGUL AND PUBLISHER

EIGHT

To HRT or not to HRT?: That is the question

My Story

Whether to use HRT is the most common question asked at my menopause conferences. It is most definitely a 'hot' topic for women going through the change.

When I first heard about HRT, I just kept visualising the word CANCER in a big bubble. I felt confused and a bit worried. And I'm used to putting all manner of drugs into my system! Progesterone... testosterone... oestrogen... bio-identical... body identical... patches... tablets... gels... Different brands, different doses. It was like a minefield. Contradictory headlines bombarded me. Might cause breast cancer; might cause dementia. Might not. Might protect against osteoarthritis. Might protect against heart disease. Might not. Talk about a rock and a hard place!

I started investigating – and while I did I read about some of the older methods used for dealing with the menopause – leeches on your genitals anyone? No? How about a clitoridectomy? (Yes, that is exactly what it sounds like...) Maybe being locked up in an asylum? Suddenly, taking a few hormones seemed like a walk in the park. However, I found that everyone had an opinion. Some friends said it wasn't natural to put synthetic hormones into your body, but having been on the pill since 15 that didn't worry me. Extolling its virtues were Andrea McLean, Lorraine Kelly,

Davina McCall and Mariella Frostrup as well as many female GPs of my age. I chose to join them and take it.

My decision to take it was based on my own personal circumstances. Osteoporosis is a constant worry for me as I already have it in my hip, so hearing HRT could protect against it getting worse was a big tick for me. Improved libido, ceasing night sweats and balancing mood swings were other big ticks. Breaking down in tears over an ad on TV, losing my temper, and nights soaked in sweat were not my idea of fun. I don't know how my family put up with me; I was having great difficulty living with me! When I heard my symptoms could go on for 15 years, I decided life is just too precious to spend it feeling like this. I deserve better. I wanted to stop barely functioning and start flourishing and I felt that HRT could help.

I considered tablets but decided against them as I heard that they can cause a higher risk of clotting. I tried the patches but I struggled to keep them on and once found one stuck to my dog's tail! So I chose the gel. With oestrogen, I take three pumps a day, sometimes another if I am not feeling too good or suffering from something like breast tenderness. Your GP will advise you on how much to use. I also take a progesterone tablet every night. Testosterone, I take one pump a day. When I had my period, I also had a coil, which gave me the progesterone I needed but I don't need that now. Twice a week I also use an oestrogen suppository as the pelvic floor is so oestrogen-receptive, as my next expert explains...

Once I suspected menopause, I went to a private gynaecologist, Dr Sara Matthews, as I just could not bear to wait to see an NHS specialist. I appreciate the cost means many women don't have this option, but for me it was worth it. She gave me a blood test to check my testosterone levels, and oestrogen and progesterone gels to use while we waited on the testosterone results. Think about it like this, the oestrogen is the fertiliser that grows, then the progesterone comes in to cut the grass down. When the blood results came back, my testosterone levels were very low, so I got some testosterone gel too. Once I got the first prescription, my own NHS GP was able to prescribe almost everything on it, so I only needed to pay for one private appointment. She also referred me to the Chelsea and Westminster Menopause Clinic – I had to wait six months for an appointment, but it was worth it to be put on their books. I go back every year for a full review.

Testosterone in a female formation is the one thing I must pay for privately. It has helped so much with my libido, energy and drive. I think it's crazy that it is not licenced in the UK. Men can get it and are also able to get Viagra so why is female libido not considered as important? Some GPs will prescribe the male version testogel to menopausal women, but it is not commonplace.

HRT was a complete game-changer for me. My night sweats went in a few days and I started to feel like Meg again. Regaining my enthusiasm, I looked forward to the day instead of struggling to get out of bed. I still find it incredible that a bit of gel can make such a difference. I also overhauled my lifestyle, exercise and nutrition as I wanted to do more than simply take something to alleviate my symptoms.

'I wanted to stop barely functioning and start flourishing and I felt that HRT could help.'

I hear horror stories of women trying to get HRT from the doctor and being fobbed off, or being told they are too young/too old for menopause; others who are told just to get on with it. Some go to one GP and get it, then go to another who takes them off it. If you are going to the doctor, my advice is to do all you can to understand the options open to you before you go. Knowledge is power. Ignorance is not bliss. Also remember that this is an incredibly personal journey. What works for others may not work for you. You need to work with your medical team and make the best choices for you - HRT or not. But if you are considering HRT, it's important you understand it - so over to my next expert, GP Dr Bella Smith.

expert view

LET'S TALK ABOUT . . . HRT

WITH DR BELLA SMITH, GP

Hormone Replacement Therapy (HRT) is a way of replacing the hormone levels that fall with menopause. It helps balance out the rollercoaster of hormones during the perimenopause and increase hormone levels when they are low post-menopause.

There are a few different combinations of hormones used within HRT. Oestrogen can be given alone to a woman with no uterus (womb) but, in a woman with a uterus, it must be combined with progestogen.

On top of this, testosterone gel or cream can be prescribed for women who have symptoms of low sexual desire and profound tiredness and where HRT on its own has not proved effective.

WHO CAN HAVE HRT?

The National Institute for Health and Care Excellence (NICE) Guidelines 2015 recommend HRT as the first line treatment for women over the age of 45 with perimenopausal symptoms and for women below 45 who are diagnosed with an early menopause. Most women can take HRT if they choose to, but it is not always available for those who have had certain hormonal cancers.

Before prescribing HRT, your health professional will do an assessment that will take into account factors like your age, weight and height. They'll discuss your personal and family history, medical factors like your blood pressure, your contraception needs and other risk factors, to ensure the benefits of taking HRT outweigh any possible risk. Alternatives to HRT, such as non-hormonal medication, lifestyle and Cognitive Behavioural Therapy, should also be discussed especially if you can't take HRT or choose not to. If you are prescribed HRT, you will have a follow up appointment three months later to ensure all is okay and then an annual check-up to discuss the treatment and whether you should remain on it longer term. There is currently no time limit for a woman to stop HRT. As long as the benefits continue to outweigh the risks you can stay on it as long as you would like. I have some patients in their 80s and 90s who are still happily taking it and still enjoying the benefits.

WHAT ARE THE BENEFITS OF HRT?

Short-term benefits are symptom relief, which can improve your quality of life day to day. HRT can reduce hot flushes, improve joint and muscle symptoms, lift mood and reduce anxiety, and improve sexual desire. Some women say HRT makes them 'feel themselves again'. There are also long-term benefits and these include maintaining bone density, preventing osteoporosis and reducing the risk of fractures. There is increasing evidence that HRT can help protect the bowels, lowering risk of colon cancer, and the heart, lowering risk of heart disease. It's also believed there may be a protective effect against dementia.

WHAT ARE THE DIFFERENT TYPES OF HRT?

You can take oestrogen in oral tablet form or transdermally.

Transdermal means 'through the skin' and describes both patches and gels. This is becoming more popular as there is good quality evidence that HRT through the skin does not increase risk of blood clots or stroke (a risk that is associated with tablets).

As discussed in chapter 5, topical oestrogen can also be used to specifically tackle symptoms affecting the vulva, vagina and urethra (see page 82).

WHAT ARE BODY AND BIOIDENTICAL HORMONES?

Hormone replacement therapy can also be divided into 'body identical' and 'bioidentical'. Body identical hormones are synthetic plant-derived hormones (oestrogen and micronised progesterone) prescribed in the UK on the NHS and are very close in nature to the hormones produced by your own body.

They are licensed, regulated, recommended in national and international guidelines, and can usually be prescribed by your NHS GP or gynaecologist as well as privately.

Bioidentical are 'compounded' hormones that are a mixture of different hormones that are not regulated or licensed in the UK. They can be mixture of oestrogen and progesterone but may also include added testosterone, thyroxine, steroids or other hormones. Bioidentical HRT tends to be expensive and is often prescribed in private clinics.

ARE THERE RISKS WITH HRT?

There may be. Research into HRT is ongoing so guidelines can change, but at the time of writing there is evidence that taking some types of HRT slightly increase the risk of breast cancer. As with all women it's important to be breast aware – examine your breasts regularly and attend routine mammograms.

HRT in tablet form has been found to increase the risk of stroke and heart disease, but there is no increased risk with transdermal HRT.

In order to make an informed decision about the risks and benefits of taking HRT, you should discuss things in detail with the health professional prescribing the drug and you should revisit your decision annually to ensure it's still the right choice for you.

SIDE-EFFECTS OF HRT

These can vary between individuals and the medications used, but progestogen can give you premenstrual symptoms such as breast tenderness, mood swings and irregular bleeding. Oestrogen can make some women feel nauseated or sick.

Side-effects of testosterone are rare but too much testosterone is linked to excess facial hair and a lowering of your voice. It's important that women using testosterone have regular blood tests to check levels. In fact, whatever hormones you are using, see your doctor if you are experiencing side-effects as the dose may need to be modified or the type of medication changed – symptoms caused by progestogen, for example, can be much reduced if you start taking a form called micronised progestogen.

In summary...

Many women suffer with menopausal symptoms that can have an impact on their physical, mental and sexual health and can alter family dynamics and their ability to work. Taking HRT can have both risks and benefits but for many women, it can be life-changing.

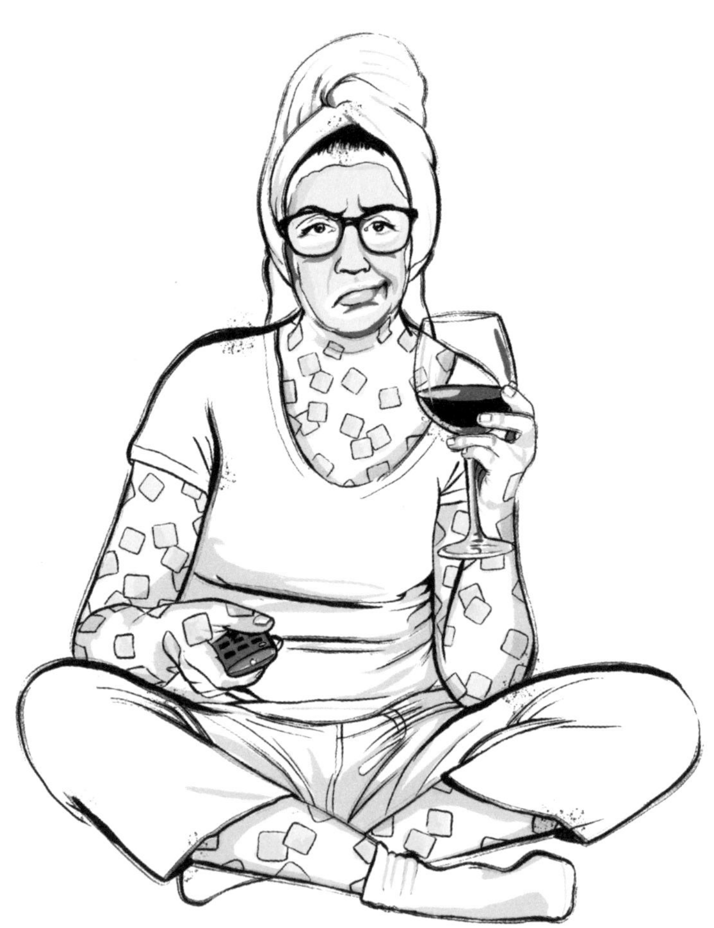

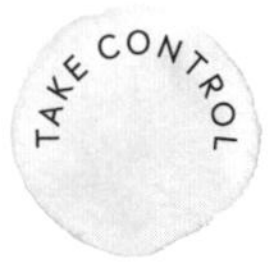

Your HRT checklist

It's important that you consider if HRT is right for you, so have a good think about things. Ask yourself questions like:

- ◯ Do I understand the different types of HRT?
- ◯ What form do I like the idea of (assuming your doctor agrees)?
- ◯ What positives might I get from using it?
- ◯ What negatives can I see from using it?

'You can't pretend it's not happening; accept it and if you need help, go and get it … I promise that afterwards there's life and it's all fine.'

DAWN FRENCH,
COMEDIAN AND AUTHOR

NINE

Hey, Doc! I need some help here

My Story

I was a bit intimidated the first time I went along to talk to my doctor about what was going on. My anxiety, low mood and forgetfulness made it challenging, and there's a lot that I wish I had known before that initial appointment.

My first tip would be to ask at the surgery if they have a menopause expert. You can check on the British Menopause Society website (thebms.org.uk) to see who is accredited and if there are any connected with your surgery. The majority of GPs don't get perimenopause and menopause training at medical school, and it is up to them to go on training courses, which is ridiculous given half the population will be affected by it at some point. Also, they have limited time per appointment so a practitioner who has an in-depth knowledge and can give you a bit more time might be a better option.

I would also advise listing all your symptoms and what you have done to try and alleviate them to make the most of the time you have in the appointment. You could take the symptom checker in the first chapter in with you (see page 23). Every woman experiences the menopause differently, so it is useful for the doctor or nurse to see what you are experiencing. It can also help them decide if any tests should be done to see if there is an underlying issue that may not be menopause-related. For example, weight gain and fatigue could be a sign of an underactive thyroid. I always make sure I have my bloods tested every year just to rule out any anything that isn't menopause-related – I do tend to worry so they give me peace of mind. I also ask for a printout of the results now – someone advised me to do that and I was glad I did. I was told on the phone everything was normal but when I got the results some showed up as abnormal. Nothing major but I was glad I asked.

Next, I would suggest that you do some research. Look at the NICE guidelines and do some reading around the menopause. You don't need to be an expert, but I found having enough knowledge to have conversations and discussions with the professionals ensured I played an active role in the decision-making around my treatment. For example, NICE guidelines state that HRT should be considered for low mood resulting from the menopause, and CBT should be considered for low mood and anxiety. Despite this, I was offered only antidepressants when I first approached the doctor, and I hear constantly from women who are given this as the only option.

I also found writing down all the questions that occurred to me and taking them with me helped (I knew menopausal brain fog would otherwise lead me to forget to ask half the things I needed to know on the day!). If you are nervous or anxious then it is also fine to take someone with you for support. They can act as your advocate if you forget anything or feel a bit overwhelmed. I often use breathing exercises to relax me.

Don't be afraid to ask for what you want. Doctors are not mind-readers and often would prefer if you were honest and direct about what you want and what you're experiencing. I have a friend who wanted counselling and just asked straight out to be referred to a therapist (she had to wait seven months but found it to be highly beneficial when she got it). You may want a referral to a menopause clinic. I find it shocking that there are so few in the UK. I was lucky enough to live in an area where there was one and found it really helpful.

Private menopause clinics may be an option to consider. The cost could rule it out, but often you only need one appointment to get what you need. Once you get the prescription, your GP is likely to prescribe the same things for you going forward. This is what I did for my first appointment - and it was worth it.

Ultimately, if you are unhappy with the support your GP gives you, you are absolutely within your rights to ask to see another GP or even change surgery.

Many women have very positive experiences with the medical profession so please don't be afraid to seek help if you need it. There are excellent doctors and nurses out there who really know their stuff and do a brilliant job. We have come a long way from the days when we were expected to just soldier on.

expert view

LET'S TALK ABOUT . . . HOW TO TALK TO YOUR DOCTOR ABOUT MENOPAUSE

WITH DR LOUISE NEWSON, GP AND MENOPAUSE SPECIALIST

It isn't always easy to approach your doctor about menopause. Sometimes it's embarrassment that makes things tricky, but often women feel uncomfortable talking to their GP about menopause because it is a natural process, rather than a disease and they don't feel they should need help getting through it. Remember having the menopause can increase risk of other diseases such as heart disease, depression and osteoporosis, so it is both okay to seek advice, and important that you do.

- Talking about your symptoms and potential solutions is going to take some time to cover so it's a good idea to ask the receptionist if there is a double appointment available when you book; the standard GP appointment of ten minutes is not very long, and can be easier for you, and the doctor, if you have slightly longer to talk. It's not always possible, but it's always worth asking.

- When you do go to the appointment it's important that your doctor considers menopause as many women find that when they go with common menopause symptoms, such as palpitations, low mood, memory problems or urinary symptoms, the doctor may focus on tackling those individual problems rather than discussing the cause. If your doctor wants to prescribe antidepressants, for example, rather than considering HRT, they should definitely be challenged as to why. There is no evidence that antidepressants improve the low mood associated with menopause.

- Even if you're considering HRT you might not walk out of the doctor's that day with a prescription. That's okay. It might not be the right time for you to start it yet, or you might want to gather more information, read some more, and then go back to discuss HRT. If you're very clued up and the doctor agrees that it's the right choice for you, then it would be appropriate to start HRT following the first consultation. Whatever happens, you should, however, leave feeling that you've be listened to and feel reassured that things will move forward in a positive way.

- Admittedly, some doctors still do have issues with prescribing HRT, which is often due to a lack of menopause training for doctors and healthcare professionals. Then it can be difficult. If you're confident, you can point them to the NICE Guidelines which state that HRT should be the first-line treatment for menopause but if you're more wary, then it can help to write to your doctor. On my website (**www.menopausedoctor.co.uk**) we have a letter template

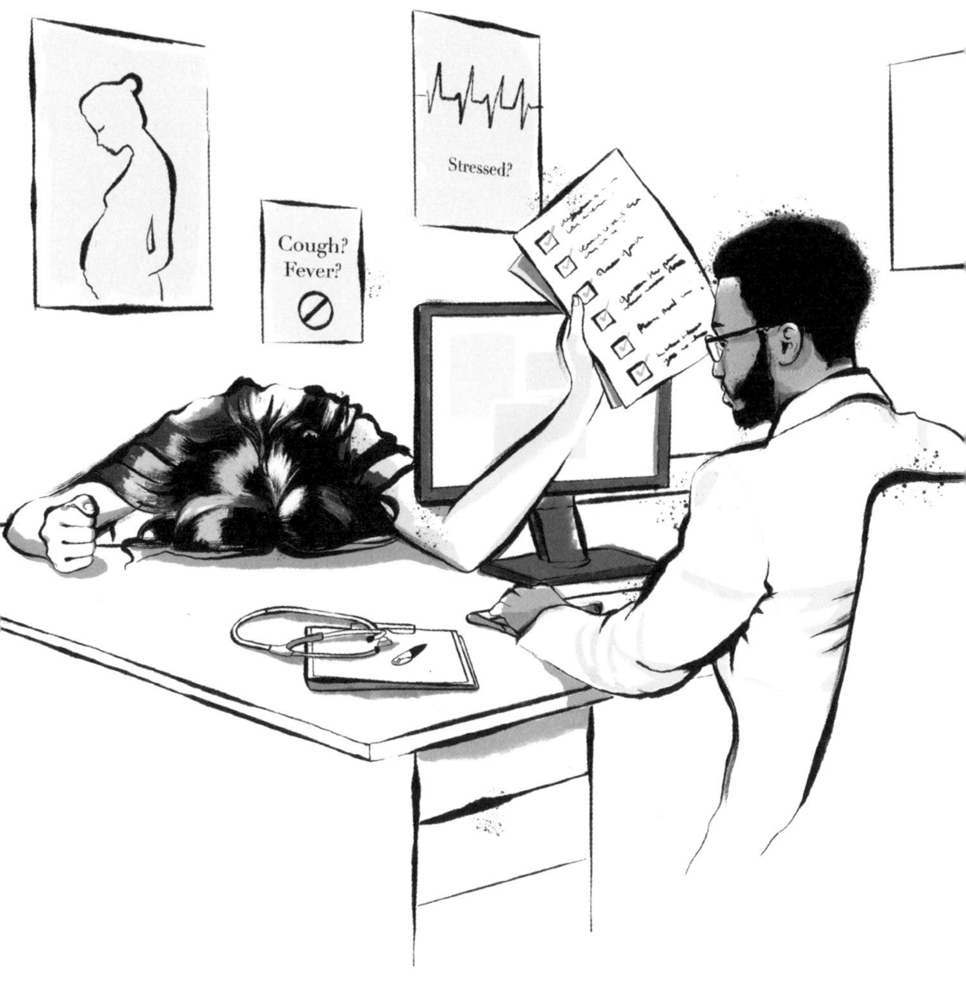
Stressed?
Cough?
Fever?

that approaches the subject in a positive but assertive way, and we've found it helps many women (just search for letter in the box on the home page). Some patients do have to see a different doctor to get results. That's okay. It's fine to ask for a second opinion.

Even if you do have the odd bump in the road, in most cases a GP is the best person to help you through menopause, but some women will also see a menopause specialist. This is most likely if you have a complicated medical history. Say, for example, you've had breast cancer or blood clots in the past, and so your normal doctor feels they don't have quite the right experience to prescribe HRT to you, then they may well refer you to a menopause specialist on the NHS. A lot of women, however, come to my clinic because sadly they've been refused HRT for the wrong reasons, and are just really struggling to receive evidence-based help. In this situation, you can ask to be referred to a menopause specialist on the NHS, but there may be a long wait, or there may not be a suitable clinic in your area (there are frustratingly few NHS menopause clinics in the UK). You can also see a private doctor without a referral from your GP, but you will have to pay.

Whoever you see, the most important thing is that you have an open-ended conversation and that you feel empowered and informed. That's what most of my work is about: ensuring women get the right help for them at a time that can feel very isolating and scary. But it is possible and you can do it.

Your pre-appointment checklist

So, you want to talk to your GP about the symptoms you are experiencing, and you think it might be perimenopause or menopause. Here are a few things to think about to help you get the most from your appointment:

- Ask if there's a menopause specialist at your surgery.
- See if you can book a longer appointment.
- Do you want to take a friend with you? See if they're free for your appointment.
- Fill in the symptom checker on page 23 and take it along, or make a note of the key symptoms for you.
- Read up on HRT and get questions ready for your doctor.
- Read the NICE guidelines and see if they mention what should be offered for your symptoms, just so you know.
- Write down any other questions or concerns.

A letter for your doctor

If you feel that you have not been listened to, and need to contact your GP again, there is a template of the letter on Dr Louise Newson's website (**www.menopausedoctor.co.uk**).

'There are lots of other things you can do if you'd prefer not to go down the HRT route; things that work with your mind and your body. But the biggest boost any of us can have when we are struggling? Love. True love is what keeps you going when none of the others will quite do...'

ANDREA MCLEAN, AUTHOR, BROADCASTER, CO-FOUNDER OF FEMALE EMPOWERMENT SITE **WWW.THISGIRLISONFIRE.COM**

TEN

Menopause au naturel

My Story

I turned to a lot of natural remedies at the start of my menopause when I didn't know what was happening to me. I was desperate, and would talk about the symptoms to my girlfriends, lots of whom do things very naturally, and they would say, 'Maybe it's a parasite you picked up in Mexico.' And I'd think, 'Well, it could be, I was swimming in those natural pools in the jungle.' So I'd do a parasite cleanse (which uses turpentine, by the way). When that didn't work, they'd say, 'Maybe it's Epstein-Barr virus...' and off I'd go see to someone who specialised in that.

I spent thousands and had so many different treatments – Kinesiology, acupuncture, Chinese herbs, breathing exercises, kundalini yoga, ice-cold baths, drinking four litres of alkaline water a day, having my tongue read, my eyes read, my stools analysed. I tried everything to tackle the symptoms. At one point, I was even working with a shaman in Hawaii. I'd lie there and she'd clear my energy over the phone from the other side of the planet – and she sent me this medallion thing for me to put water on and it would cleanse the water I was drinking each day. This all makes me laugh now I know what I really needed was a bit of gel that costs the NHS a few pounds, but at the time I had no idea. Don't get me wrong; this wasn't the fault of any of the practitioners – they didn't know I was going through menopause. Nor am I saying that natural remedies don't work for menopause. They can and they do. In fact, there are many remedies out there that can naturally balance hormones and reduce the effects of symptoms. And even though I managed my menopause medically, I still use natural remedies as part of my approach. I use CBD oil to help with anxiety and crystals for detoxification. I use colloidal silver to boost immunity and protect against germs. I also enjoy matcha powder with almond milk. It is packed with antioxidants and calms my mind and relaxes me. I find it also helps reduce my menopausal brain fog.

Other friends of mine, however, have embraced the holistic side of menopause a bit more - like the wonderful and wise Lynne Franks who was kind enough to share her experience with me:

Lynne's story

My menopause came on fully in my early 50s, when I was firmly ensconced in a California lifestyle, where I thrived in the constant sunlight, worked out on the beach every morning while watching the dolphins play, meditated regularly, cycled all over my area of Venice Beach and ate healthy food.

Because of my lifestyle at this point, it was natural for me not to drink coffee or tea. I had regular liver detoxes and drank lots of water in the heat. I didn't drink alcohol because Californians didn't, as we drove everywhere.

So, by some kind of luck, I found myself living a lifestyle I would advise for anyone experiencing a tough menopause, but you don't have to go to Los Angeles to eat well, keep away from alcohol and coffee and drink lots of water – all of which I would recommend alongside exercise that you truly enjoy. I danced my way through my menopause – and beyond! I investigated taking HRT privately but decided against it. I put on some yam cream for a couple of months and basically just cruised along with a new life of no more monthly bleeding and pain, with far more energy, a strong libido and most of all, a much clearer mind.

The menopause for me represented my passage to Wise Woman, where I can use my experiences, good or bad, to show others how to create a life of purpose and joy. Now in my early 70s and living in Somerset, I believe this period of my life is the best yet. I watch my grandchildren blossom alongside my own children being great parents. While ensuring my own wellbeing with the right supplements and nutrition, I have moved to a small English market town where I have opened my SEED sustainable eco-hub, café, lifestyle store and online community – and I still dance!'

So, what if you would like to follow Lynn's example and manage your menopause naturally? For that, I'll turn you over to my next set of experts to explain what's on offer:

“

‘The menopause for me represented my passage to Wise Woman, where I can use my experiences, good or bad, to show others how to create a life of purpose and joy’

expert view

LET'S TALK ABOUT . . . MANAGING THE MENOPAUSE NATURALLY

WITH CAROLINE GASKIN, HOMEOPATH AND NATURAL HEALTH PRACTITIONER

My personal choice is always to do things naturally, and through my work I see many women who want the same. There are a number of reasons for this, some women are sensitive to synthetic hormones like the birth control pill and the morning after pill and don't want to take HRT. Or it may be that HRT is contraindicated for other more serious health reasons. Others try HRT but feel some side-effects – bioidentical hormones can, for example, create excessive anxiety or sleep issues for some women, but you can use natural remedies to create balance.

HOMEOPATHY

This is based on the belief that the body has an innate intelligence and can cure itself. Tiny amounts of natural substances from plants and minerals are given to stimulate the healing process. Homeopathy is not to be confused with herbal medicine, Ayurveda or aromatherapy, where much larger doses of plants and herbs are used.

Homeopathy has many remedies for menopause symptoms, such as Pulsatilla for irregular cycles, Sepia for grumpiness and feeling indifferent to life, and Lachesis for heavy flooding. However, while you can buy homeopathic remedies in health food shops, it's best to work with a homeopath to find the remedy that's right for you, as choosing the best one relies on a little bit more than just ticking off physical symptoms. As a homeopath I'm looking at 'how' it is, and what's changed. Sepia, for instance, is good when the menstrual cycle gets shorter. It's good for headaches that come before the period. Lachesis can help if you wake with a headache. Both remedies can be good for hot flushes, but in the consulting room, the Lachesis patient will talk very fast, telling me everything at great speed, the Sepia patient will seem apathetic, not bothered and might be irritable answering my questions. It's important to get the right remedy for you to get the best results.

BALANCING HORMONES

Many glands are involved in balancing your hormones and at menopause the thyroid, adrenal glands and hypothalamus, as well as ovaries, need support. These glands get mixed messages due to environmental toxins such as fluoride, chlorine and bromide, so reducing exposure to external chemicals can help. Drinking filtered or spring water and choosing a mattress made from natural fibres can be small but vital steps in reducing toxin exposure and can make a significant difference.

Another tip is to take homeopathic tissue salts, as these are universally available. Kali Phos is good for anxiety and feeling edgy, and Mag Phos is good for muscle cramps, headaches and period pains. Ferrum Phos can help anaemia and Calc Phos can help achy bones and tiredness. You can take these alongside conventional medicine but consult a practitioner and get some tests if you don't see any improvement after a couple of weeks.

ADRENAL SUPPORT

The adrenal glands need particular attention. We still make oestrogen after menopause - just not as much - and our adrenals take over the role of producing it. They also produce the hormone cortisol that we release during stress and as we've said before (see page 20), the menopause happens at a time when stress can be high. The need to make more cortisol, combined with the role of producing oestrogen, can mean our adrenals struggle and even minor situations suddenly seem out of proportion. It's common to feel like a madness has taken over and that life is completely out of our control, but balancing the adrenals can help.

I often prescribe homeopathic remedies for adrenal function like Black Eyed Susan for busy people and Macrocarpa for extreme exhaustion.

Nutrition and lifestyle choices such as restorative yoga, skin brushing and hot and cold showers also benefit adrenal health.

Adrenal glands are involved in our response to allergens so it's no surprise that skin issues and food sensitivities can also show up at menopause. In perimenopause I got a rash from a new face cream and then over-reacted to an insect bite and the Chinese herbs I was taking. Work was busy and I was travelling and it was just too much for my adrenal glands

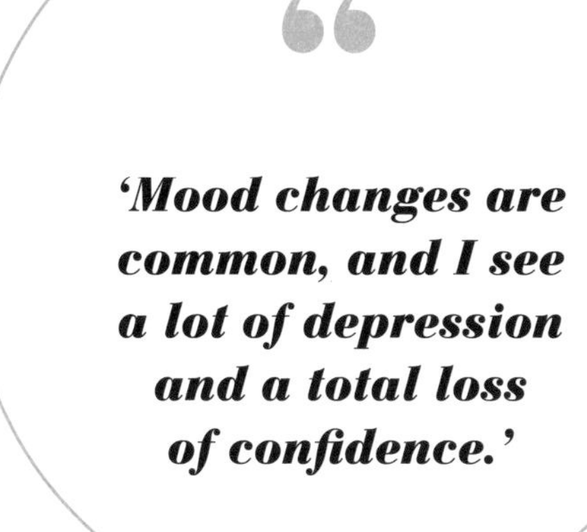

'Mood changes are common, and I see a lot of depression and a total loss of confidence.'

to cope with. Some relaxing craniosacral treatment for stress and Nux Vomica, a homeopathic remedy to support liver function, sorted me out and may also help you.

Magnesium is also important for our stress response. It's best absorbed through the skin using a magnesium chloride spray oil or by taking an Epsom salt bath. Magnesium helps to balance blood sugar, soothe nerves and draw up minerals essential for bone health. The latest studies show that stress and anxiety can take a toll on our bones, something we definitely don't need at this time.

Lastly, many women notice less tolerance to alcohol. Red and rosé wine tend to stimulate adrenal glands more than other alcoholic drinks. Try natural wines or organic wines without sulphites.

PROTECT YOUR LIVER

The liver processes toxins and breaks down hormones, so reducing alcohol, sugar and refined carbohydrates will help liver function. Supporting the liver is fundamental to look after breast health and reduce insomnia, hot flushes, headaches and night sweats.

Many women take milk thistle to support liver function, and essential fatty acids help too. Dandelion is another great tonic for both liver and kidneys.

EMOTIONAL SUPPORT

Mood changes are common, and I see a lot of depression and loss of confidence. I prescribe flower essences for emotional issues and to promote wellbeing. Woman Essence, by Australian Bush Flower Essences, is a blend to help with focus, ease worries and balance female hormones, while Purifying Essence helps with drug side effects, detox and with clearing negative thoughts.

You may also find yourself grieving for times past, for children you've lost or children you couldn't have. Regrets also surface about relationships. We also experience isolation and self-blame. These are big issues that need support. Talking helps and I might refer clients to a spiritual healer, bereavement counselor or creative writing class as extra ways to work through things. Menopause is a huge transition on many levels.

During my own menopause, I found my thoughts going back to a time in my 20s when, as a young mum, I'd experienced a big shock; I realised that now my children were older and fending for themselves, the protective maternal part of me could finally relax. Insights like this helped me transition and appreciate how far I'd come. I believe this is the gift of menopause: the wisdom that comes can be a tool to support others.

expert view

LET'S TALK ABOUT . . . HERBAL HELPERS

WITH AILSA HICHENS, NUTRITIONAL THERAPIST

There are many herbal remedies indicated for tackling symptoms of the menopause and, if you can't or don't want to take HRT, finding the right remedy for you can be a good way to help you get your symptoms under control. However, tempting as it might be to buy up the whole menopause aisle to try and find a solution, you don't want to go from zero to 'taking everything I found in the shop'. Instead, have a look at the suggestions below and pick the herb that you think will work best for the symptoms that worry you most. Take at the dose suggested on the label for at least eight weeks and see if you notice a benefit.

ASHWAGANDHA

This root is one of the Ayurvedic herbs. In Sanskrit, its name basically means 'horse smell', so you might guess that it's not the nicest herb to take, although once it's tucked away in a capsule, you won't really notice. You will notice the effects though. Folklore says it's supposed to give you the strength and virility of a horse, which is a bit of a curious concept, but in reality it's amazing for helping you cope with stress and supporting the adrenals during menopause.

AGNUS CASTUS

Sometimes called chaste-tree, this is good for women at all stages of their hormonal life. During menopause, it particularly helps balance that really crazy feeling where your periods think you're a teenager again – perfectly okay one month, light the next and then suddenly flooding like someone's killed you in your bed!

BLACK COHOSH

This herb tackles some of the symptoms that bother women most at menopause – hot flushes and night sweats. There is a bit of a dispute about its exact mechanism of action; we know it seems to have a similar effect in the body to oestrogen, but interestingly, it doesn't actually increase oestrogen levels. Black cohosh also seems to have a positive effect on dopamine and serotonin receptors and may fight that 'I'm a bit low but I can't quite put my finger on why', feeling that can hit at menopause. Only buy brands that carry a THR (Traditional Herbal Registration) mark, which says it's come from a reputable source and is delivered at a safe dose (all the ones sold in places like Boots or Holland & Barrett will have this) as some small studies have shown problems of toxicity with unlicensed black cohosh. It's also not recommended for anyone with liver problems.

GINKGO BILOBA

Many people report that their memory gets a bit hazy as they get older. It's a curse for both sexes and it's usually a question of age rather than hormones. That said, one thing women talk to me about a great deal in clinic is that fuzzy-headed feeling, sometimes accompanied by a low mood, and Ginkgo biloba (the leaves are what is used to create both tinctures and capsules) is something I often use for gently lifting this feeling. A study in 2014 found that taking a Ginkgo biloba supplement also increased sexual desire in menopausal women, likely thanks to its positive effect on blood circulation. At a time when women are frequently struggling with lack of confidence in their own bodies, vaginal dryness and low libido, feeling more sexy counts as a real win.

MACA

This has been used for many years as a female health tonic and aphrodisiac so, if low desire is your most concerning symptom, it can be worth trying - although libido is not the only thing it helps. There's also evidence of maca helping with hot flushes, night sweats, insomnia and vaginal dryness. You can use the root as a loose powder to put in smoothies or in capsules. Maca is generally a very safe herb, but I have had the odd client who felt a bit weird when using it, so do keep an eye on things and stop if you feel a bit out of sorts.

SAGE

This helps with temperature regulation. One trial in Switzerland found that within four weeks, about half of the women taking it found that their hot flushes had disappeared. If they carried on for eight weeks that went up to 64 per cent. Women also see improvements on mood and brain fog as sage is known to be very good generally for memory.

SEA BUCKTHORN

The oil from this plant is a source of omega-7, an essential fat that keeps the mucus membranes healthy, meaning it might help with vaginal dryness. One study on women taking 3g a day for three months showed clear improvements on symptoms of vaginal atrophy.

FIND YOUR DREAM TEAM

While you can buy many alternative remedies over the counter in health food shops, it can be good to work with a professional to ensure you're getting the best treatment at the right dose. There are a few different natural therapists who can help you on your menopause journey including:

ACUPUNCTURISTS

Acupuncture uses very fine needles inserted into specific points of the body to balance the body and treat specific conditions. You can find a qualified acupuncturist via the British Acupuncture Council **acupuncture.org.uk.**

HOMEOPATHS

Correctly pinpointing the right homeopathic remedy for a person is not as easy as just looking at the main symptom; the client's personality and exact presentation also matter. Working with a homeopath will ensure you get the right remedy for you.

You can visit the British Homeopathic Association at **britishhomeopathic.org** to find one.

MEDICAL HERBALISTS

Medical herbalists use plant-based remedies to help treat symptoms and causes of illness. They have studied some form of medicine and have the same diagnostic powers as a GP, and base remedies around herbs where the traditional use of the plant is backed up with clear science.

To find one visit **nimh.org.uk**.

NATUROPATHS
Naturopathy is the study of natural medicine. A naturopath won't just treat one symptom; they will look at your whole health picture and work with that. They may use herbal or other remedies and lifestyle changes in treatment. To find a qualified naturopath visit **gcrn.org.uk**.

NUTRITIONAL THERAPISTS
Nutritional therapists work to improve health using dietary means. This may mean the food you eat and/or the use of supplementation to tackle symptoms and correct deficiencies behind health concerns. Visit **BANT.org.uk** to find registered therapists.

Sticking it to menopause

Another treatment that might help menopause is acupuncture. It might look a little scary with all those needles, but perhaps, surprisingly, it's a super gentle and natural therapy to balance menopause symptoms – and it's proven to work too. One recent Danish study, for example, found that after five weeks of acupuncture, symptoms including hot flushes, night sweats, sleep disturbances and emotion problems were lessened.

In Chinese medicine, it's thought that menopause symptoms occur due to a lack of yin energy caused by day-to-day living, stress, work and all the rest. The idea is that acupuncture helps re-establish the regular flow of energy.

'[Menopause] signals a new beginning, rather than the end. So I treat my body as I would a car about to go on a new journey; keep it running smoothly by putting the best fuel you can afford in it. Do all you can in order to keep the gears running smoothly and for God's sake don't leave it in the garage gathering dust!'

TRISHA GODDARD, TV PRESENTER

ELEVEN

Eat to beat your hormones

My Story

It might sound a bit odd that someone who used to live on cigarettes, rum and recreational drugs is now almost fanatical about nutrition. I've realised now that what you put into your body can make a huge difference to how you feel, and I'm so much more aware of what I put in my body and how it fuels me. I think it's a shame that most GPs and menopause clinics don't talk about how important good lifestyle is and simply talk about medication. I want to be the absolute best I can be through all sorts of approaches, and now know that what I eat affects my mood, gives me energy and protects me against disease – if I make the right choices!

So far, my cholesterol and blood pressure are fine, but my mum died of a stroke, which could mean hereditary factors are against me, so I try to eat as well as I can. I have talked about my fear of osteoporosis, so I take a calcium supplement and eat a lot of green leafy vegetables such as kale, as they are naturally high in calcium. And if I am being honest… as well as health, there is my vanity. I gain weight more easily than I used to and I feel so down when the scale starts swinging up and my 'menopot' starts to increase. I want my clothes to look good on me.

I'll tell you a bit about my food and drink intake in a typical day. I stress that I am not a nutritionist and I don't say it's the right plan for everyone... it's just what works for me.

When I get up, I have two pints of warm water with fresh lemon juice squeezed into it. I continue to sip on another three litres of water throughout the day as I feel awful if I get dehydrated. I use my favourite bottle and fill it from my filter jug - that saves money and is also better for the environment than buying bottled. I also find if I drink a lot of water, I can avoid those hormonal acne break-outs that take you back to your teenage years (so frustrating - wrinkles or acne should be the rule - not both!). I am completely teetotal now and look back at my alcohol-filled days with a bit of incredulity. I don't know how I functioned with the amount of booze going through my system.

I eat a plant-based diet and tend to eat mainly in the evenings with my drinks keeping me going throughout the day. Some disagree with this saying you should eat more regularly, but I find it works for me. I became vegetarian when I was eight - adamant that I would never eat anything that had a face - and went fully vegan in my late 40s. People often say, 'But what about protein?' It is actually quite easy to get sufficient protein through a vegan diet - legumes, soy-rich food, oatmeal, quinoa, buckwheat, nuts and many seeds will give sufficient protein. It's also a lot easier now as all the supermarkets carry such a wide range of vegan foods.

Tonight, I am having vegan sausages with mashed potato with olive oil instead of butter. I would never win *MasterChef* – this is about as creative as it gets. I often get meals delivered, which may sound a bit of a luxury, but everyone who knows me knows I am such an awful cook, it's worth it.

I have also eliminated dairy, gluten and sugar from my diet. I used to be guilty of grabbing unhealthy snacks when I was out and about so this was a real mindset shift as most snacks contain one or more of these. I now just carry some nuts with me. Eating out can also be a bit of a minefield as the portions are often so big – so much bigger than they were a couple of decades ago. I often just have a starter rather than a main course. I am lucky in that I never really had a sweet tooth. A treat for me is a few blueberries, some peanut butter and some coconut yogurt.

I also have vitamin B12 shots monthly as it is very common for menopausal women to become B12 deficient. B12 is essential for energy and making serotonin, which controls your mood. I am prone to low mood and find this really helps me. It also helps me sleep. To ensure I get my other nutrients, I also take one of my Menoblends from my range. This is a food supplement containing vitamin C and B6, calcium and complex B vitamins including folic acid, niacin (vitamin B3) and pantothenic acid (vitamin B5). That's the science – but basically, they are all designed to alleviate menopausal symptoms in one way or another.

“

‘I gave up drinking alcohol over a year ago and it’s been a game-changer! I also notice a real difference if my diet isn’t great or I’m not drinking enough water.’

I find eating healthily so much easier than doing enough exercise. I genuinely enjoy eating healthy food and if I do fall off the wagon then I really feel it. Before, I’d then give up and binge for days – but now I don’t beat myself up. I just jump right back on it.

That’s my plan, but I’m not saying all of you need to go vegan to feel good – so, let’s hand over to my next set of experts to talk about what you can do.

expert view

LET'S TALK ABOUT . . . FOOD AS MEDICINE

WITH ROB HOBSON, REGISTERED NUTRITIONIST

During menopause, choosing foods with some specific ingredients can help with menopause symptoms like hot flushes, or counteract long-term effects on bone density, heart health and metabolism. The risk of heart disease increases after menopause, but maintaining a healthy weight and adopting a Mediterranean way of eating, which includes an abundance of plant foods, has been proven to support the health of your heart.

Here's what to include:

PHYTOESTROGENS

Found in plants, these substances have a similar, but weaker, effect to human oestrogen in the body, and they may help to relieve symptoms such as hot flushes. Foods rich in phytoestrogens should be eaten daily and include beans, pulses, nuts, seeds, berries and soy foods (such as tofu, tempeh and miso). It can take a few months for the benefits to be felt and some women respond better than others, but stick with it as these foods promote good health in many other ways. Whether or not you should consume soy if you have a family history, or personal experience of breast cancer, has been controversial. However, current expert advice is that eating 1–3 servings per day of soy foods as part of a balanced diet is fine, but soy isoflavone supplements, which contain much higher concentrations, are best avoided.

OMEGA-3 FATS

Found in oily fish, nuts and seeds, omega-3 fats reduce inflammation in the body, and research suggests they may help with hot flushes and night sweats. If you're following a plant-based diet, you may want to take a vegan omega-3 supplement as the fats from plant sources are not as easily used by the body as those found in fish.

PROTEIN

Muscle mass declines during the menopause, impacting on metabolism and weight. Maintaining a greater muscle-fat ratio will keep your metabolic rate fired up and help tackle 'meno-middle' and protein is essential for this. You need at least 50 grams of protein each day so try to include it in every meal (including breakfast): 25 grams equates to a fillet of chicken or fish or half a can of cooked beans, pulses or lentils. An egg contains 5 grams of protein.

CALCIUM

Vital for bone health. Our bone stores start to deplete from our mid-30s and loss accelerates at menopause. Include 2–3 calcium-rich foods in your daily diet, such as dairy products, fortified plant drinks, green leafy vegetables, tofu, seeds, pulses and dried fruit (bread is also fortified with calcium in the UK).

VITAMIN D

Helps the body absorb calcium. In summer we make this from exposure to sunlight, but in the winter months, take a supplement of 10mcg.

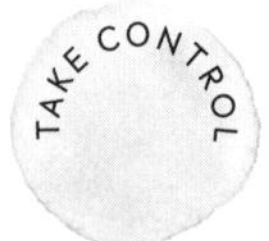

A Meno-friendly plan

What does all that look like day to day? Here's a simple three-day plan to give you some ideas.

DAY ONE

Breakfast:	***Lunch:***	***Dinner:***	***Snacks:***
Porridge made with plant or dairy milk, topped with chopped dried apricots and a few nuts and/or seeds.	Mixed bean salad with tomato, onion and feta cheese.	Salmon with brown rice, spinach and red peppers.	A handful of nuts. A piece of fruit or a handful of berries.

DAY TWO

Breakfast:	***Lunch:***	***Dinner:***	***Snacks:***
Bircher-style muesli or overnight oats with yogurt and fruit.	Sardines on wholegrain toast with edamame beans.	Chicken and cannellini bean stew with spinach and broccoli.	Greek yogurt with fruit. Peanut butter on celery.

DAY THREE

Breakfast:	***Lunch:***	***Dinner:***	***Snacks:***
Smashed avocado and feta on sourdough or wholegrain toast.	Tuna and quinoa salad with tomato and cucumber.	King prawn stir-fry with soba noodles, kale and mushrooms.	Hummus and crudités. Handful of edamame beans.

expert view

LET'S TALK ABOUT . . . IS THE GUT THE MISSING LINK?

WITH SARAH GRANT, NUTRITIONAL THERAPIST

The health of the bacteria in the gut has been making news in the health world for a while now. Research has linked a healthy balance of bacteria in the gut to better mood and reduced anxiety, and, while we're still investigating how it plays a role, there's also a belief that the bacteria may play a role in the menopause experience too.

When oestrogen has done its work in the body, it's sent to the liver where it's bound up as a signal to your body that it should be excreted. However, some bacteria in the bowel can cause that oestrogen to become unbound and re-circulate into the bloodstream. If you have too much of that bacteria, too much oestrogen may recirculate and, at a time when the body is already out of balance hormonally, this extra oestrogen could potentially exacerbate imbalances between progesterone and oestrogen and make symptoms worse.

Looking after the gut bacteria balance could be an extra piece in the menopause wellness puzzle. So, how do you do it?

The first, and most important tip, is to eat a 'rainbow' of plant foods every day - mix up the types and colours you eat. Plant foods - fruits, vegetables, wholegrains, herbs, spices etc - contain fibres and polyphenols that help the good bacteria to flourish. Fibre from plants also help keep the bowels working well, helping you pass old oestrogen out of the system faster, so limiting the time bacteria can act on it. Good hydration is also important for keeping things regular.

Prebiotic foods contain substances that feed good bacteria and help them to thrive - they include many plant foods with special mentions going to mushrooms, oats, barley, garlic, bananas and Jerusalem artichokes. Also, look for probiotic foods that naturally supply more good bacteria to the bowel. These include foods like kimchi, sauerkraut and natural yogurt. Kefir is a drink that seems to help get the bacteria through the stomach to where it needs to be, so perhaps give that a try too.

While ideally you want to get all the nutrients you need from a healthy diet, if you're busy that doesn't always happen. Also, during menopause there are some key vitamins and minerals your body may use more of, or deplete more quickly, and so supplementing can be a good insurance policy. Up next, Ailsa Hichens looks at what's particularly important in any supplement you choose.

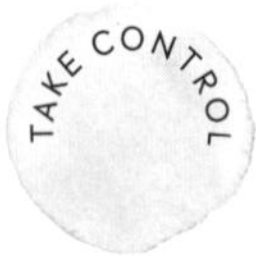

Additional insurance

WITH AILSA HICHENS, REGISTERED NUTRITIONAL THERAPIST AND HEALTH COACH

You need good quality B-vitamins. These are the vitamins that we tend to associate with providing energy, but they are really, really important for women going through the menopause as they help support the stress response. As oestrogen production from the ovary declines, your adrenal glands start picking up the slack and it's important that you're supporting them. Particularly look for brands that contain the methyl forms of folate and vitamin B12 as these are easiest for your body to use.

As Rob said, vitamin D is essential – and in a supplement you should look for vitamin D3 which is the form your body uses. We can make this from sunlight in summer, but the older you get the less good your skin is at creating it. Vitamin D is important in the menopause years for bone health, but also for blood sugar balance and the prevention of diabetes.

You also need vitamin C. This does so many things – it's antibacterial, antiviral, antifungal, an antioxidant and it stimulates production of collagen. But it's also involved in handling stress.

Minerals are also essential particularly magnesium which is important for hormonal health, and it is another substance used up very quickly when the body is tackling stress.

I also look for iodine, which is very good for thyroid function – the thyroid can need support right now.

Lastly, for women of this age, I also like supplements to contain a substance called diindolylmethane (DIM), which is really helpful for helping the metabolism of oestrogen.

That might sound like you're going to rattle, but choose a good quality multivitamin and mineral that contains them all, rather than take them all individually.

'I've always needed my gym time
but never more so than in menopause.
It's literally become a tonic for me.
It might sound counter-intuitive but
building up a sweat, however you
choose to do it, will also help with
the hot flushes.'

MICHELLE HEATON, SINGER AND AUTHOR OF *HOT FLUSH: MOTHERHOOD, THE MENOPAUSE AND ME*
(MICHAEL O'MARA)

TWELVE

Let's get physical

My Story

People tell me I look fit and strong and assume that I am also an exercise junkie. But outside impressions can be deceptive and nothing could be further from the truth: I am just lucky to have been born with a muscular physique – literally, my mum told me I was born with muscular quads. The reality is, I hate exercise and will find any excuse not to go. I am essentially a lazy person. Give me a boxset and a comfy couch over working out any time! At the height of my menopause I simply could not be bothered; I was so demotivated and lacking in energy. I gained weight and became more lethargic. So, exercising became even harder – it's a real vicious circle.

Over time, though, I've realised that the benefits of exercise to me are immense. And I find focusing on them helps my motivation. So what are the benefits?

Well, I like to look good and being toned helps with that. I gained two stone when I was menopausal, and it was really tough to get rid of it (weight loss is WAY harder in your 50s than in your 20s), but I find exercise helps to keep it off. I do a lot of public speaking and know I feel so much more confident when I wear clothes that show off rather than hide my figure.

Avoiding my osteoporosis getting worse is another benefit. I do weight-bearing exercises for 45 mins a week with a trainer to help specifically work on my bones. I also do Pilates as that also helps. Like everyone, my risk of cardiovascular disease increases as I get older, so I make sure I do exercise that gets my blood pumping. I like the odd body combat class; it makes me feel fierce and in control. I also do HIIT (high intensity interval training), which is good when I'm busy as I can just download the exercises and do them in the house for 15 mins a day. And I run – I am not a great runner but the Couch to 5K plan helped (you can find it on an app and online), as did doing it with a friend.

The lift in my mood from the happy hormones that flood your body during exercise is another benefit. I particularly get this buzz if I can exercise outside. I really enjoy walking my dog Ziggy – being outside and saying hello to people and their dogs is a great start to my day. It's important to find something that suits you. I don't like team sports, but I know people that love to have games of volleyball and football. Also, I did join a gym that was great but quite a distance from where I lived. I have now joined a less flash one that is less than a five-minute walk from my house, so it is much more accessible and easier to fit workouts around my life. If I can't be bothered now, I remind myself that I ALWAYS feel better after. However hard it is to get up and go, I know that once done I never, ever regret it. Never once do I jump in the shower after a workout and say 'Oh I wish I hadn't bothered.'

So, how do you find what motivates you? Well, maybe it'll come from the following list of benefits from trainer Christina Howells, or the suggested workout from another of my favourite trainers, Lucy Wyndham Read.

expert view

LET'S TALK ABOUT . . . THE BENEFITS OF EXERCISE

WITH CHRISTINA HOWELLS, PERSONAL TRAINER

It sucks, right, when things change out of our control? But while ageing is inevitable and menopause is a natural transition that brings with it challenges, declining fitness and health are not necessarily part of either of them. So, flip the script, address what needs to be done, make a plan, and positively define your new chapter.

While during much of our life exercise may mostly be linked with aesthetic goals, during menopause its potential to reduce our risk of major diseases and live a fuller life is far more important. Our health and quality of life, are to a large extent, driven by our lifestyle choices, and exercise is an invaluable form of protective medicine that all of us have access to.

The most life-threatening concern post-menopause is heart disease, which is the biggest killer of women in the UK. Menopause does not cause heart disease, but a decline in oestrogen does alter physiology in ways that increase your risk of it. However, the vast majority of cases can be prevented through protective lifestyle factors such as exercise.

Weight gain is a common topic during menopause, but it's also not a direct symptom, and more likely a result of ageing, diet and inactivity. However, a decline in oestrogen does influence the shift of fat towards the midsection. Being overweight and, specifically, having abdominal obesity, increase the risk of diabetes, high blood pressure and high cholesterol, which all in turn further increase the potential of heart disease. The more active you are the easier weight is to control.

Exercise can also help beat meno-fatigue. Inactivity breeds inactivity – the less we do the harder it is to motivate ourselves and the more tired we feel; conversely, the more active we are, the more likely we are to feel energised and uplifted.

And what about your bones? There is a direct relationship between the lack of oestrogen after menopause and the development of osteoporosis, but bones are just like your heart and will stay strong if you give them work to do; when your muscles move, they pull on your bones which strengthens them. To strengthen muscles and bones, you need to move them against resistance with exercise like weight training or expose them to impact from walking, running or aerobics.

For all of these benefits being active, ideally for 30 minutes or more, most days of the week, is recommended. In addition to moving more daily, you also want to be specifically working your muscles 2–3 times a week with resistance training using your own body weight, bands or weights , dynamic yoga and Pilates.

expert view

LET'S TALK ABOUT . . . HOW TO EXERCISE

WITH LUCY WYNDHAM READ, YOUTUBE FITNESS EXPERT AND PERSONAL TRAINER

Exercise can become your best friend during menopause. It can work wonders on how you feel and the physical benefits you get from each workout are endless. So, here's how to get results.

To strengthen your bones, you need to do body-weight training, which means you don't need to use equipment so you can do it at home, outdoors or at the gym. Exercises include press ups, lunges, squats, star jumps or just jogging on the spot, all of which use the weight of your body as resistance.

Looking after the heart means cardio training; this is any form of exercise that helps to get your heart rate up so you are feeling a little out of breath. You could try walking briskly, running, cycling or even just walking up and down the stairs.

'A phrase I love to remember when thinking about joint health is that "motion is lotion".'

For joint health, we want to stay nice and supple, and simply being active and doing exercises that have a full range of motion, like walking and swimming, help to keep things fluid. A phrase I love to remember when thinking about joint health is that 'motion is lotion'.

Pretty much every exercise also helps mental health by reducing stress, anxiety and depression. Having a positive mind keeps everything on track. Yoga and stretching can help, but all exercise helps reduce stress hormones and raise the level of feel-good hormones.

And finally, you'll want to fight that dreaded menopausal weight gain. A great way to take control of this is with exercise. If time or cost is a factor, even a short home workout that uses major muscle groups and dynamic moves like star jumps, or skater lunges will help. These engage more muscles per move than static exercises and so help increase your natural calorie burn. Over the page is a short workout to help you do this.

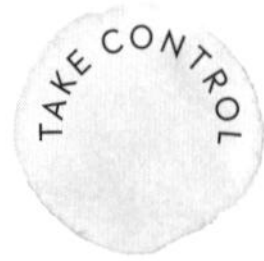

The 5-minute menopause workout

You can do this at home, outdoors or at the gym. Each exercise takes 1 minute, so you will do about 5 minutes in total. Do it once in the morning then also later in the day if you can, or repeat it twice and turn it to a 10-minute workout. In that short time you will have worked your whole body!

1. ***Standing elbow to knee crunches***
This exercise helps to shape your waist and warms you up, as well as working your balance and flexibility. Stand upright with your feet shoulder-width distance apart. Your arms are bent with elbows in line with your shoulders, palms facing forwards. Now, in a controlled manner, lift one foot off the floor aiming to get your knee to hip height, then at the same time, bring the opposite elbow towards the knee by rotating slightly through your waist. Hold then take your knee slowly back and forwards for 1 minute, then do the same on the opposite side.

2. ***Step back lunges***
This exercise strengthens the bones in your lower body, tones your legs and bottom and increases your calorie burn. Start with your feet wider than hip-width distance apart, with your body straight and tummy muscles pulled in. Take a deep step behind bending the knee. Hold for a second then push back up. Repeat on the other side, then alternate from one leg to the other for 1 minute. If you find it hard to balance then do this next to a wall and put your hand on to the wall to support you.

3. ***Ladder run or march***
This exercise improves your heart and bone health, burns off excess body fat and tones your arms. Simply run or march on the spot with your arms lifted up and mimic the movement of climbing up a ladder.

4. ***Squat to punch***

This exercise helps to reduce anxiety and stress, increases cardiovascular health and shapes and sculpts the lower body. Start by standing with your feet slightly wider than shoulder-width distance apart. Bend your knees as if you are about to sit down on a chair. Hold for a second then come back up (be sure not to let your knees go over the line of your toes). Repeat eight times. After the eight squats, remain standing and punch your arms out straight in front for eight counts. Go back to the squats, then the punches, and keep alternating for the minute.

5. ***Press up***

This exercise strengthens the bones throughout your upper body, lifts the bust, tones the arms and works your core. Here are three variations of a press up – use whichever you feel most comfortable with. A box press up starts on all-fours on the ground. Bend the elbows and lower your upper body slowly to towards the ground (this is ideal for a beginner).

If that's too easy, from that box position push your hips forwards so now you are doing a ¾ press up, and again lower your upper body towards the ground.

If this is still too easy do a full press up where you have your legs straight out behind you and balance on your toes. Again, lower your upper body gently to the floor.

Whichever you choose, repeat for 1 minute.

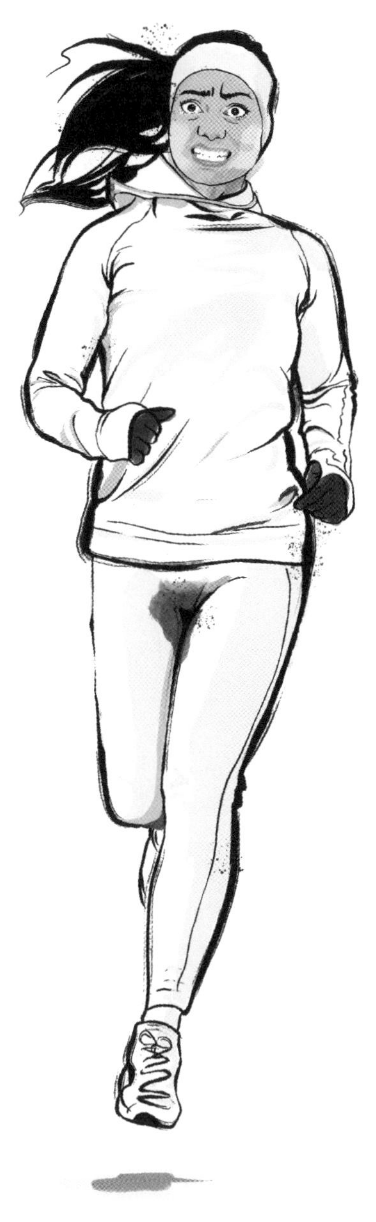

'Our mothers were largely silent about what happened to them as they passed through this midlife change. But a new generation of women has already started to break the wall of silence.'

TRISHA POSNER,
AUTHOR AND JOURNALIST

THIRTEEN

It's Good to Talk

My Story

Talking is my survival mechanism; it's how I get through the bad times and the good, and I've always found it easy to pour out my feelings and emotions. I talk to my friends and family. I talk at numerous events including my own menopause conferences. I even talk to strangers in the hair salon. Emotional pain is not something that should be hidden away. When I started menopause it was no different; conversation was how I coped. Being open and honest can be frightening, but reassuring yourself that it is okay to not be okay at this time in our lives can help. It isn't a weakness to seek help – it is a strength.

I have tried professional talking therapy once or twice, but I always preferred talking to people I know and I have some great friends that I can talk to about anything. I have memories of sitting in a local restaurant talking for hours to a friend about all the things we had tried to alleviate our menopausal symptoms. To me, that was the best therapy ever – and it was completely free. However, I understand that for many women, a professional is sometimes needed. The experience, skill and empathy of a therapist may help you in a way that friends and family can't, and I hear of many women who have gained a whole new perspective on life through talking to a professional.

'Catastrophising' is one of my negative thought patterns and one that's difficult to alter. I would obsess about public appearances and imagine people looking at me and me totally messing up. Talking to others has helped me with this and has helped me build a 'can do' attitude. I also used to catastrophise about the osteoporosis in my hip, envisioning becoming bedbound and a burden to all. Now my thought pattern is more focused on what I can do to prevent myself getting worse; I no longer focus on the limitations of getting older, and instead I focus on what I can do.

Thankfully, mental health is no longer a taboo topic. High-profile celebrities and even royalty now talk openly about challenges with depression. People understand more now, and the good old British 'stiff upper lip' and 'grin and bear it' attitudes are fast becoming relics of the past. It is also good that menopause is now to be taught in schools; if children understand what is happening to their parent, it can help them deal with it. I resent like hell that I didn't know what menopause meant until I was crash bang in the middle of it all. The more we talk about it then the more we normalise it and reduce the associated stigma.

Talking and raising awareness is what I am all about and I know you want to talk about menopause too; my website had over 700k views in its first year. When I was on *Women's Hour*, we were inundated with questions. I have run two conferences with over 400 attendees and have enjoyed talking to everyone at them – and the feedback is that everyone loved having an outlet to talk and found it really reassuring. I also have a podcast series where I talk to experts, which I find so useful. Many women contact me afterwards to say how good it was to hear professionals give evidence-based information to help them, and it makes me feel empowered to know that I am doing something to help other women.

Twenty years ago, you never heard the word menopause – even five years ago it was more whispered about than talked about. I am passionate about addressing this and making it as common a topic as pregnancy. But I admit sometimes that isn't so easy, which is why I asked my next expert for some advice.

expert view

LET'S TALK ABOUT . . . STARTING CONVERSATIONS

WITH DIANE DANZEBRINK, MENOPAUSE CONSULTANT, COUNSELLOR AND CAMPAIGNER

'It's good to talk' is perhaps not a surprising statement coming from somebody who spends the majority of her time listening to and supporting women, but it's also true that talking is not always easy during menopause.

If you don't really understand what's going on it can feel impossible to start a conversation about it with those closest to you.

Often, that's where I come in, as someone who can listen and explain. The most common phrases that I hear on a daily basis are: 'I feel like I am going mad', 'I feel so alone, and 'I have lost me'. As a woman who experienced a very dark time as a result of my own menopause, I can really empathise with those statements, and finding somebody to talk to who really gets it is absolutely key.

When you want to talk about menopause with family or friends it is worth taking some time to prepare; it's important to have some basic facts to share with them and arrange a time to sit down together and talk about it calmly. Ask your partner, family members or friends if they would give you the time to explain how your symptoms are affecting you and also share what they could do to help you through this time in your life. Clearly, the conversation will be different depending on whether you are talking to adults or children and will depend on whether your children are teenagers or younger. Our loved ones often feel confused during menopause as they don't understand it, and anything you can do to normalise the conversation will help them and you. If talking to your partner family or friends is just too much for you right now, write things down and send each of them a note explaining how you feel; you could enclose some factual information about menopause to help them understand more about it. Most important of all, let them know how they can best support you through this time in your life.

Talking also helps you feel more in control during menopause. If you're with friends, family or trusted colleagues and have a hot flush, why not simply say that's what's happening? By being proactive, you take ownership of the situation and you might be surprised by the empathy that you receive; after all over 50 per cent of the population will experience menopause and you never know, you might just help a friend or colleague too.

Probably the least discussed symptoms of the menopause are the urinary and vaginal symptoms, and you may be thinking, 'Well, how can talking help those?' But these are not just physical symptoms. The debilitating effects of vaginal pain or discomfort, the physical changes to our genitalia and the resulting effect on our most intimate relationships with

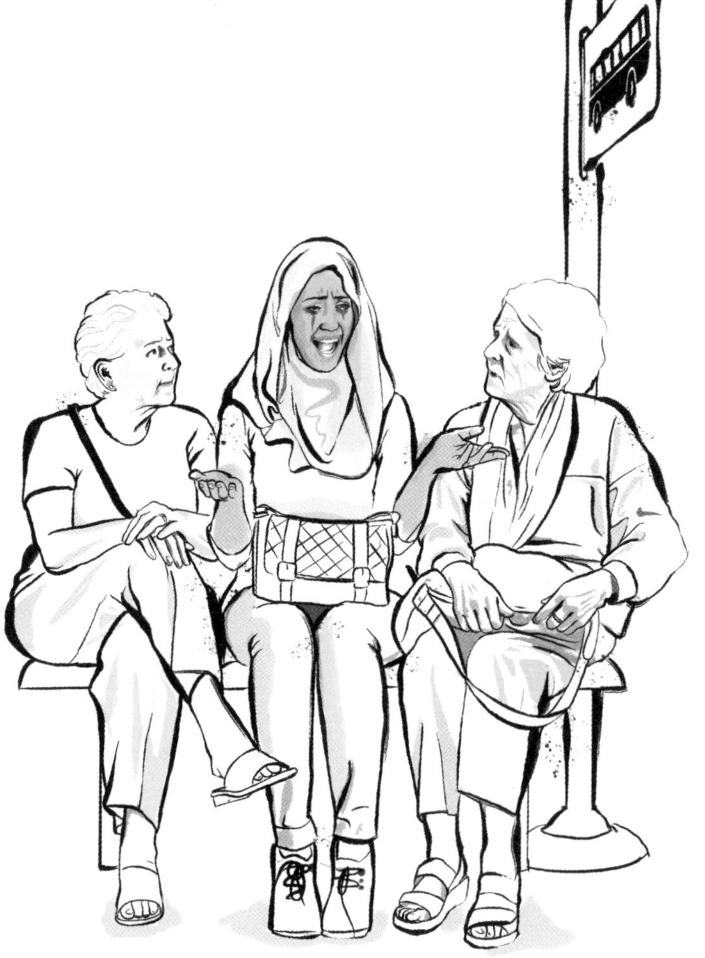

ourselves and partners can be emotionally devastating. Having somebody to talk to about that can be lifesaving and shouldn't be underestimated.

Often it is possible to physically see the weight lifting from the shoulders of women going through menopause once they talk – I see women recognise that they are not going mad, that it is not their fault and that there is hope for the future. Don't miss out.

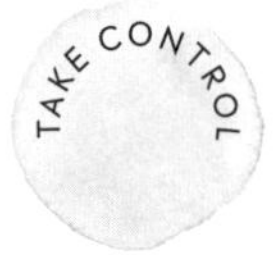

How to find someone to talk to…

When choosing a friend to talk to, you should pick someone that will be supportive – but support can come in different ways. If you just want to offload, your super-practical friend who likes to give advice is not the best person to speak with that day, instead, pick the one who just sits and listens. If you do want advice on how you're feeling or to help you move forward, get your go-go-go friend on speed dial immediately.

If you choose professional therapy, then make sure your therapist is a registered member of BACP (British Association for Counselling and Psychotherapy). Also think about what form would suit you best. There are many options; most therapists will do phone, FaceTime, Skype or email sessions if you prefer. There isn't a 'best' or 'right' way; it's about choosing what suits you. If, in time, you feel you simply don't connect with a therapist, it is fine to choose a different one.

Online forums can also give support and it's amazing how therapeutic simply talking to other people in the same situation as you can be. One of the biggest is at menopausematters.co.uk. You may want to check out if there are any menopausal meet ups near you – menopausecafe.net organise some and I am working on setting up my own groups in the near future.

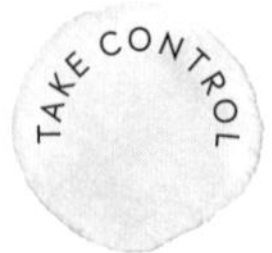

Start writing

If you don't feel comfortable talking to others, writing about how you're feeling, also known as 'journaling', can be a really great way to let out feelings and clear your head. It can also help you feel more positive and, because it switches on the creative, right-hand side of your brain, it may even help you come up with solutions to some of the niggling menopause challenges you face each day. Here's how to make it work for you:

- **Get a beautiful book and pen**
  You want to feel like you're investing in yourself when you journal, and writing in a book you think is pretty, that revitalises you, or just makes you feel good and special in some way will help that. A decent pen that works well will make it all the more enjoyable.

- **Don't be an editor**
  This isn't a school essay – don't worry about spelling or sentence structure or whether it all flows together. You're just letting out your thoughts and feelings, so just set an amount of time to write and just scribble down anything that you're feeling. It might be good, it might be bad, it might be odd words and not even full sentences – but just let the words flow.

- **Think of what you can learn**
  Don't just write about the negatives that are in your head; after you've let things out for a little while, try and examine your feelings from different angles. Consider what you can learn from experiences and think about where to go next.

- **Finish on a high**
  Just before you put down your pen, write down three things today that you feel grateful for or that made you feel happy, or that went well. They don't have to be big wins like a promotion or a pay rise; think about small wins like noticing how fast your dog's tail wags when you came home can be enough. The more you look for positives in life, the more positives you see, and it can really help change how you're feeling.

expert view

LET'S TALK ABOUT . . . FEMALE FRIENDSHIP

WITH JO WOOD, MODEL AND ENTREPRENEUR

Female friendship is so important when you are going through major life events like menopause. I first met Meg in the mid-90s and we became instant friends; she is a Pisces, I am a Pisces and we were both married at that time to rock stars. We have a lot in common. As the years have gone on, our friendship has only got stronger and we have always been there for each other through good times and bad. It's good to know that I have a great female friend in Meg ... and I cherished our friendship during menopause and now. I also spoke to my mum about what was happening. I think it's great that women talk about menopause, especially with each other, because it's one of the most natural things in the world.

Every woman since time began has gone through the menopause so it should be something that we talk about openly. I didn't have a difficult menopause, but if I had, I would definitely have spoken about it more.

“

‘I felt really isolated when the menopause hit – like no one really understood me. I joined a couple of online forums and it was great to be able to vent about my symptoms and realise I wasn’t alone.’

'Every workplace needs to be better informed about the perimenopause and menopause, and how symptoms can profoundly affect the health and wellbeing of its female employees. Currently, most employers tend to focus on maternity leave and flexible working hours for parents with young children, but not every woman will have a child. Every woman will have a menopause.'

LIZ EARLE, MBE

FOURTEEN

Stand by me

My Story

As well as hearing from menopausal women, I often hear from significant others in their lives asking for help in supporting someone they love or work with. I will always remember one man who showed up at one of my events. He sat quietly at the back and, at the end, he confided that his wife was going to come but felt too overwhelmed to attend so he came to see if he could get any information. I could empathise with his wife and was quite emotional at her husband's efforts to help her. That's where I got the idea for this chapter – the idea is that you can hand it to the significant others in your lives to give them ideas on how best to support you.

So, if you've just been handed this... what can you do to support the woman in your life? Educating yourself on the menopause is key – understanding why she may be acting like she is. You don't need an encyclopaedic knowledge but a base knowledge, perhaps by reading the first chapter in this book (see page 15), is useful. Once my friends and family found out that the swinging moods, hot flushes, fatigue and low libido were typical and not related to anything they were doing themselves they started to relax.

Maybe you're reading this off your own back because you know someone who you think might be menopausal and are not sure how to broach it with them. I wish someone had talked to me earlier. I'd advise anyone who is seeing someone suffer to perhaps casually drop it in to conversation or use a more direct approach – you could save them from years of distress. If you don't feel comfortable opening a conversation, then perhaps you can get your hands on some leaflets from the doctor's surgery or even print articles out from the internet. I will be forever grateful to that woman I met at AA who gently took me aside and said it might be worth me reading up on it. She gave me her number and told me to call her if I wanted to chat about the menopause. I couldn't wait to ring her. To me, that is a good friend.

My mum died before I started the menopause and I miss her so much. She was from a generation that did not talk about such things, but I know that if I had opened the conversation, we would have talked through it and she could have told me about her experiences. I hear of many women whose experience mimics their mothers.

Needing a bit of kindness is something all menopausal women probably have in common. Small gestures such as filling a bath and putting some candles on can make someone feel special. Someone once changed my bedding when I was exhausted – lovely clean fresh sheets felt so good. Friends suggesting walks helped – a chance to talk and the fresh air lifted my spirits as the endorphins from the exercise kicked in. Think about what sends your person over the edge – if she can't cope with big family gatherings maybe pick up the slack and do the organising. Doing something as simple as a bit more of your share of the housework on the darkest days can help. These small tokens of affection are very important as most women hitting menopausal age also start to feel a little invisible, isolated and rather lonely.

Listening is something else that costs nothing and is so under-estimated. Giving full attention and putting gadgets like mobile phones away will obviously help. Simply asking the question: 'Tell me what I can do that will make things easier for you?' can be a good opener. I was not sleeping, and the snoring of my partner made it worse. When he asked me that, I said, 'Please sleep in the guest bedroom a few nights a week,' and he did. It made such a difference; a good night's sleep is what most menopausal woman crave. Maybe they don't want to talk, and it is then just a case of reminding them you will always be there when they do.

If your sexual partner is going through the menopause and their libido has fallen, then you may be feeling rejected. Please remember that this isn't a reflection of you. During the menopause the vagina can shrink both ways and become paper thin, and sometimes it is agony to get a finger in let alone anything bigger. Imagine someone vigorously sandpapering your genitals then wanting to have sex – it feels a bit like that. The best way to support your partner through this is to accept it and look at alternatives to penetration and go at her pace. Lots of lube can help (see page 70), and remember a tongue is much more gentle than other parts of the body! Although she may not want to be as sexually active as before, your partner is likely to still want to feel cared for and appreciated. Maybe a night in with a film and a takeaway, a day out somewhere, a nice lunch... anything that makes them feel special and creates a little intimacy.

It is important to be more tolerant and patient. On the other hand, you can't let anyone consistently act in a rude or abusive way towards you. You need to have your boundaries on the types of behaviour that you will and won't accept. Helping someone going through a bad menopause can take its toll. Make sure you have support in place so that your own wellbeing doesn't fall by the wayside. Practising self-care is important for both of you.

If you are in a position at work where you can create or influence the support given to menopausal women, then it is worth perhaps getting a focus group together and asking their opinions. I know of one workplace where a 22-year-old woman and two middle-aged men put a menopause policy together – the only thing of use in it was to offer women a fan! Conversely, one very enlightened workplace I know runs monthly menopause meetups with expert speakers to support it. They also have an internal chat room for menopausal women to support each other. They also actively support the women, allowing them to work from home if they have had a bad night and allow flexible hours so women don't have to hot flush their way through the rush hour. There is a true recognition of how valuable these women are to the workplace, and measures are in place to ensure they can keep giving their best in a supportive environment. If you don't already have a menopause policy, now might be a good time to start developing one.

With half the population experiencing the menopause at some point in their lives, it is highly likely everyone will know and be affected by someone going through it. Everyone needs different support as they will all experience the symptoms in a different way and will have different ways of trying to deal with it. I needed a little boost from time to time. I needed patience and friendship. I wanted to talk about it and not be brushed off. It was important that the lines of communication stayed open.

And there is light at the end of the tunnel. It does not go on forever and there will be highs as well as lows as you move onto the next chapter in your lives. Getting through the bumpy ride together can really strengthen your relationship, whether it is partner, friend, family member or colleague.

“

‘Everyone needs different support as we will all experience the symptoms in a different way and will have different ways of dealing with it. There is light at the end of the tunnel. It does not go on forever.’

Ten things not to say to a menopausal woman

Here is a light-hearted guide to what NOT to say to your significant other/friend/colleague when they are menopausal:

- 'What's wrong with you? Has your HRT patch fallen off? *Hahahaha...*'
- 'Are you taking part in Movember?'
- 'Let's just put the heating up a bit.'
- 'Wow, you have gained weight... oops I mean umm... you look SO well.'
- 'My granny is going through that menopause thing too.'
- 'Sorry there is no chocolate or wine in the house.'
- 'Let's go out clubbing til 3am.'
- 'Don't you think you are maybe over-reacting?
- 'I just sailed through it – no problems at all.'
- 'Calm down!'

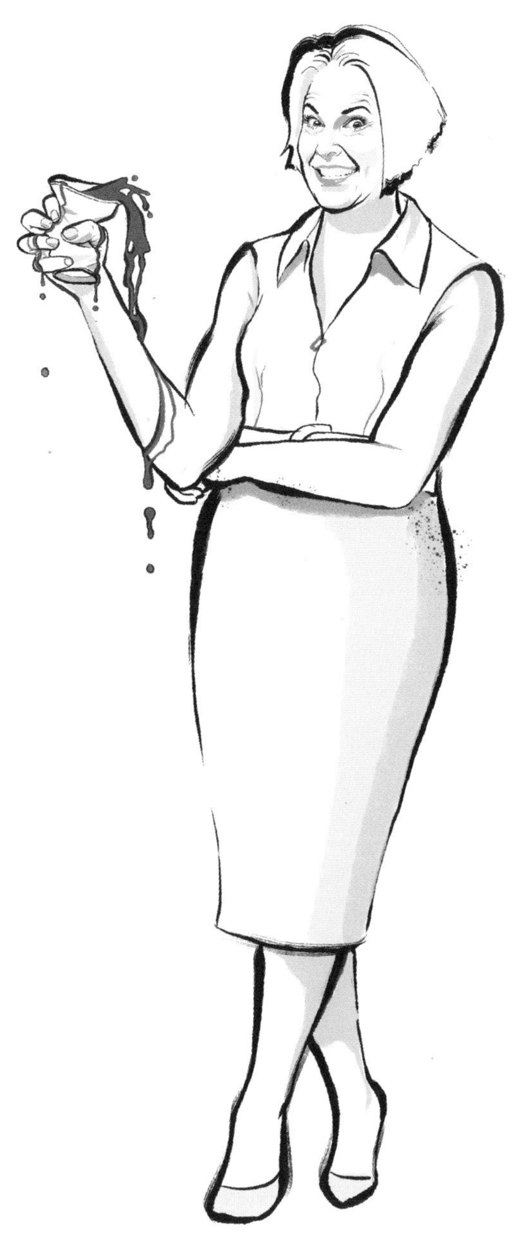

expert view

LET'S TALK ABOUT . . . SUPPORTING MY MUM

BY ANAÏS GALLAGHER

I didn't know what was going on with my mum at first. I just noticed that her moods and behaviour were getting more erratic. She had always been way more emotional than me – but now it was off the scale. I remember mentioning that I liked a particular lentil bake. I came home from school and there were seven of those bakes in the fridge – one for every night. I was laughing and she got mad then burst into tears. This started to happen all the time. She was so unpredictable: fine one minute then crying, then angry. She'd talk about me being a hormonal teenager – but I was nothing on her!

It caused issues with family dynamics at first – in a family, what one person experiences affects everyone. But then I started to try to understand. I talked to a friend at school whose mum was also menopausal and when I was able to 'label' it, I felt a bit better. I realised she was still my mum but needed some support and help from me. It was time for me to step up a bit; I felt our relationship shifted a bit as I started to look out for her. I stopped taking the moods personally, realising it was menopause and not me causing them. I did little things like make her a drink or go for a walk outside with her as I knew that helped. A trigger for her moods would be the state of my bedroom so I made more effort to keep it tidy.

The advice I would give other children who have a parent who is going through the menopause would be:

BE UNDERSTANDING

Read up a bit on the menopause so that you know what to expect and can start to have a bit of empathy of what it must be like (it sounded a bit like permanent PMT to me!).

TALK

Maybe your mum hasn't told you yet - you could open the conversation by saying someone at school's mum is going through menopause and ask if she is. It's easy to feel uncomfortable with conversations but I found the more we talked the easier it got.

DO LITTLE THINGS TO HELP

Making a cup of tea or going for a walk can help. Also, my mum was more tired than normal, so I did a bit more round the house. My mum and I always had a good relationship, but I think going through this together really strengthened it. It changed our relationship and moved it more to adult-adult rather than parent-child. We talk about anything and everything now and I love seeing how she has come out the other side and provides support to so many other women.

I still hope they have found a cure before I get there though!!!

expert view

LET'S TALK ABOUT ... HANDLING THE MENOPAUSE AT WORK

WITH DIANE DANZEBRINK, MENOPAUSE CONSULTANT, COUNSELLOR AND CAMPAIGNER

One of the hardest places to open up is at work. I can guarantee that after every menopause awareness presentation that I deliver in the workplace there will be a queue of women waiting to speak to me privately. Usually it transpires that those women have been with their organisations for a long time but now find themselves unable to cope with their workload in the way they usually would.

If that sounds familiar, work can feel like a very lonely place and opening the conversation with your employer, a daunting prospect. Thankfully, more and more employers are recognising the need to understand menopause and how offering support to staff will help them retain valuable team members. But how do you seek out that support when you are feeling nothing like your old self?

MAKE A PLAN

If you are considering speaking to your employer, make sure you prepare. You may be the first person to raise this subject so it's worth getting some information together and thinking what adjustments your employer could consider that would work for you. This allows them the opportunity to go away and decide what they could do to help.

TALK TO OTHERS

Find a friend, or identify a colleague or colleagues you can discuss your menopause with. This could be the menopause champion, if the organisation has one, or simply somebody you know who will understand what you are going through.

Starting a support group, either in person or via a social-media platform, can be very beneficial, and having the opportunity to share what has helped you with others can be very rewarding.

PRACTISE SELF-CARE

Let's be clear – self-care is not selfish; we cannot be good for others unless we are good to ourselves. Modern life is fast and sometimes feels overwhelming, but it is vital that you prioritise yourself so that you can continue to give your best to all aspects of your life, including your work.

'I am now in menopause . . . but I feel at ease with whatever will come. Not because I am strong, but because this is a part of life. It is nothing to be feared.'

ANGELINA JOLIE, ACTRESS

FIFTEEN

Too soon!

My Story

Most people will experience the menopause in their early 50s, but it can happen earlier – and often with very little warning. I went through it in my late 40s so probably a little bit younger than the average, but it could not be classed as an early menopause (or to give it the proper name 'premature ovarian insufficiency', which happens before the age of 40). Early menopause can be triggered by the removal of the ovaries (a 'surgical' menopause), or, a 'medical' menopause from radiation therapy, chemotherapy or certain medications. And sometimes it can just happen naturally and the cause will never be uncovered.

There is very little knowledge and information out there about early menopause, but what I have learned through research is that it is way more complex than simply having menopause a bit early. I believe every woman should be fully informed about what it means, especially about their reproductive choices and long-term health before any treatment, especially if you want to have children at some point. I hear time and time again of women who had hysterectomies and did not realise they would go straight into menopause with unnecessary suffering, often for years, as the result. It is incredible to think that no medical professional thought of telling them before or after the procedure, or how to manage afterwards.

I support the Daisy Network, which is a charity dedicated to providing information and support to women diagnosed with premature menopause. They are a great support network for the 1 per cent of women under 40 who will find themselves in this situation. I invited a woman from the Daisy Network, who experienced early menopause in her teens, to talk at one of my conferences. Her story had many of the audience in tears. She was so embarrassed that she didn't want to tell her mum and continued to ask for tampons then just threw them away. At school she pretended she was having periods so she could feel the same as everyone else. She no longer has the choice as to whether to have a baby or not, which devastated her.

Here in the book, we hear a similar story from Bethany Harrold who also underwent early menopause. I'm so pleased she agreed to tell us her story as I know how much hearing from someone who has gone through the same situation can help. Over to Bethany:

Bethany's story

I was 14 going on 15. I loved school, going out with my friends and spending time with my family. I had dreams and future career goals that I was desperately excited to achieve. I was just a child, a young girl with no idea what I was about to face. The mood swings, hot flushes, and fast weight gain seemed to appear somewhat overnight, and at that time it all added up to what I believed was just teenage hormones, being at 'that age'. I had no reason to think any different... until my period stopped.

A quick trip to the GP led to blood tests, ultrasounds and a complete invasion of my personal life. And after what felt like a lifetime, we had a result. My parents were devastated with the diagnosis and made the decision to transfer to private healthcare for a second opinion. From there, I had more pots to pee in, more blood tests, another ultrasound or two, until finally we had my second and same diagnosis... premature menopause. Now, before this moment, menopause to me was a phase of life that was for the older generation, something my grandmas were experiencing at the time, and something that just 'happens' when a woman reaches a certain age.

I sat there next to my parents as the gynaecologist started to explain my diagnosis. My parents both sat crying next to me, my mind fogged over, and I felt everything I had, all of my future dreams, start to slip away. I remember the doctor say in the most sympathetic voice: 'Don't worry, when it comes around to you wanting children, come back to us, there are lots of different options.' I had not thought about motherhood before that day, I was only a child myself, but at that moment and for years after, it became all I could think of. It became all I wanted and I made a lot of mindless judgements, wasting a lot of money on pregnancy tests hoping that they were wrong, and that the random stomach aches, and sickness were more than just in my head.

Following on from my diagnosis, I received a prescription for Celeste, a contraceptive pill to take until told otherwise.

I never really understood why I was to take this medication, especially as my school friends started taking the same tablets for the 'right' reason. I carried on anyway as my mum expressed how they were very important to me and my health, especially my bones. Within weeks the symptoms seemed to disappear with just the odd hot flush here and there and life seemed to be carrying on as normal, until one day, my best friend announced at school that she was pregnant. Something clicked and I became what I can only describe as jealous, angry and broken-hearted. The tears wouldn't stop as I came to realise what my diagnosis meant and the life I wouldn't be able to have as others would.

I made the rash decision to stop taking my medication, deeming it completely pointless, which made my symptoms return with a vengeance. My mood swings became worse as I pushed more and more people away, constantly battling with people who were only trying to help me. The hot flushes came back and led me to regularly standing in the rain hoping to cool down before I passed out; something that did happen once in the toilets whilst I was at school. I had no care for anything anymore; school became an unwanted chore, going out and seeing my friends became harder, and I really believed that I was completely alone in this, and no one else could ever understand.

My childhood was over, and being only a young teenager, I had never actually thought anything about my future other than what I wanted to be when I was older; paramedic, police officer, zoologist... the list went on and on over the years. But the sad thing is, I gave it all up when I became desperate to fill the void inside me, something I believed only motherhood could fill.

“

‘It took me a long time to realise what my diagnosis was doing to me, to my physical and mental health, and even my relationships. Menopause did not just change my life, it controlled my life’

As I grew older, more and more symptoms became apparent. Lack of sex drive? No, it would be better described as 'the no sex drive switch', meaning one moment I was completely up for it but it could be only a matter of minutes and it just switched off! This was something that men seemed to struggle to understand. I became embarrassed by my illness, and as the years went by, my symptoms never seemed to disappear. Was this due to my bad habits? Or was this normal for menopause? I was lost and confused, my mental health deteriorated and I became suicidal, struggling to see any future for myself.

It took me a long time to realise what my diagnosis was doing to me, to my physical and mental health, and even to my relationships. Nine years after my diagnosis, after years of no medication or treatment, I finally made the right choice in returning to the GP to get the help I needed. And once again, after a few more blood tests and an ultrasound, I am doing what I should have done from the beginning and am looking after myself.

Menopause did not just change my life, it controlled my life, but I finally feel like I have taken the control back. In March 2019 I started an organisation to raise awareness and to fundraise for UK charities surrounding infertility, including the Daisy Network. I also now volunteer as their Social Media Manager, helping others like myself, to ensure that no one feels as alone and confused as I did. Please come talk to us if you need to.

expert view

LET'S TALK ABOUT . . . EARLY MENOPAUSE

WITH MS TANIA ADIB, GYNAECOLOGIST AND MENOPAUSE EXPERT

Few women expect to get hot flushes when they haven't yet celebrated their 40th birthday. The menopause can be tough whatever your age, but when it happens to women in their 20s and 30s it can be a particularly isolating and confusing experience. Even women in their early 40s who have menopause a bit earlier than normal can feel let down by their bodies. As a gynaecologist who specialises in both menopause and female cancers, many of my patients are younger women who are going through a process that they simply hadn't envisioned happening to them for many years. It's vital that women experiencing premature menopause have a good understanding what is happening to their bodies, and know that there is help and treatment out there.

Early menopause – or to use the medical term, premature ovarian insufficiency (POI) – is defined as a loss of normal function of your ovaries before you are 40. It affects approximately 1 in 100 women but a small percentage – around 0.1 per cent – will develop premature ovarian insufficiency by the age of 30.

DIAGNOSING EARLY MENOPAUSE

A lot of women first come to my clinic with symptoms that perplex them – mood swings, brain fog, vaginal itching and pain during intercourse. These symptoms aren't always due to the early menopause, but when they're mentioned, premature ovarian insufficiency is certainly on my radar, and it's something I'll start investigating.

Other women know exactly what is happening to them and why because they have gone through cancer treatments such as chemotherapy or have had their ovaries removed. They may have medical conditions or genetic factors, such as Turner's syndrome, Fragile X or lupus that are associated with early menopause. However, for most women who find their ovaries are not functioning as they should, there won't be a clear explanation of why it is happening.

If premature ovarian insufficiency is suspected, a series of blood tests will be used to check the levels of the hormones and FSH (Follicle Stimulating Hormone). High levels of this is one of the markers for menopause as your body makes more of it in an attempt to kick-start the ovaries. Getting the diagnosis can initially take women aback, after all, it's not something any of us usually plan for. If you do enter early menopause, it's an emotional journey as well as a physical one, so be kind to yourself at this time.

FERTILITY AND EARLY MENOPAUSE

Some women discover they are in premature menopause when

they are trying to get pregnant; it is much more difficult for women who have started to go through the menopause to conceive. In 5–10 per cent of women where ovarian insufficiency happens without explanation (rather than a woman who has had a full removal of her uterus and ovaries), there may be some function still in the ovaries and they may be able to conceive, but the majority won't.

If you haven't had children yet and wish to, or if you have not completed your family, a diagnosis of POI can very hard to come to terms with, but remember, there are options out there to explore, including using donor eggs and in vitro fertilisation (IVF). There's more information on this in the next section (see page 224).

Even for women who did not plan to have children or who have completed their families, finding your fertility has ended is difficult to process. Many women talk of this as a loss as their choice been taken from them. Each woman will experience this uniquely and there isn't a right or wrong response.

LONG-TERM EFFECTS OF EARLY MENOPAUSE

Once a diagnosis of premature menopause has been made you should decide with your doctor a strategy to manage your symptoms. I really urge women not to take a stiff upper lip attitude to this, or minimise the need to tackle it. The fact is, early menopause that is left untreated can have potentially serious long-term effects such as osteoporosis and heart problems – it's also been linked with increased risk of dementia, Parkinson's and depression. This might sound alarming, but the good news is, we can offer treatments which can considerably lower these risks, like HRT.

Women with premature menopause can be assured that the controversies that surround the use of HRT (studies have linked it to a small increase in the risk of breast cancer in older post-menopausal women) do not apply to them. The research has shown that women who take HRT for premature menopause before the age of 50 have a lower risk of breast cancer compared with controls. All the evidence points to the fact HRT is safe and beneficial to treat premature ovarian insufficiency.

SURGICAL MENOPAUSE

Some women may have to undergo a hysterectomy that includes removing both ovaries. Without the ovaries, your body cannot produce oestrogen, so the operation means your body will go into a surgically induced menopause. This can mean quite a sudden introduction to the symptoms of menopause almost overnight. Hormone treatment with oestrogen and testosterone is very important here to optimise health.

If you do need this surgery, it's important to prepare. In the weeks beforehand, make sure you eat well, with lots of healthy and wholesome foods. Enjoy time with friends who make you laugh and who you can connect with emotionally. Exercise, such as walking and yoga, will help prepare you, body, mind and soul. Learning mindfulness is something I also recommend; it's a good way to help counteract any fears and stresses of surgery. Try it by focusing on your breathing for five minutes - simply slow down and be present in yourself. Learning mindfulness before the operation will be helpful afterwards to deal with hot flushes and other symptoms which you might find distressing (see also page 54).

On a practical level, make sure you have cool clothing ready to help with the night sweats - you may feel cold one minute and hot the next. It would be a good idea to stock up on ice packs and keep extra sheets by the side of your bed - you may need them if a night sweat leaves them drenched.

NON-HORMONAL TREATMENTS

So, what happens if you've had a cancer that is linked to oestrogen, meaning you can't take HRT, or simply would prefer not to? In these cases, menopause specialists can treat each symptom individually. Hot flushes can be dealt with via a low dose

'My lack of understanding led to me underestimating the impact of the menopause on my life.'

antidepressant. A specifically designed exercise programme can alleviate the risks of osteoporosis, while non-hormonal moisturisers and lubricants can be helpful in easing the discomfort of vagina dryness.

Also, don't rule out new technologies: vaginal laser treatment uses a fractionated carbon dioxide laser to boost collagen and improve dryness and lubrication, while radiofrequency, another non-hormonal treatment, can improve incontinence and help restore confidence.

YOUR MENOPAUSE, YOUR WAY

Whatever you decide after having a diagnosis of early menopause, never forget there is help out there. Finding a specialist with particular expertise in the menopause will make a big difference to your life and getting the treatment you need. Remember, the menopause – whatever age it comes – is a time to think about what you really want out of life. Once your menopause management plan is in place, it's time to live your life and really enjoy it.

How to seek help for early menopause

It's very important to seek advice if you think you might be going through early menopause, particularly if you want to consider options that might preserve your fertility.

- Fill in the symptom checker on page 23 – it's just as valid for you as older women.
- Investigate your family history. While it's not a given that if your mum had an early menopause you will too, there can be a link – so, if possible, ask her questions about her experience.
- If your doctor doesn't mention it, bring up the subject of early menopause and why it's concerning you – and see what they say.
- If they do consider it an option you should be offered blood tests to check your hormone levels and possibly an ultrasound to examine your ovaries and egg reserves.
- If you are diagnosed, you're probably going to feel a lot of the shock and upset that Bethany experienced (see page 213), so speak to the Daisy Network or check out their website at **daisynetwork.org.uk**. They can offer help, support and advice.

expert view

LET'S TALK ABOUT . . . FERTILITY

WITH DR LARISA CORDA, OBSTETRICIAN, GYNAECOLOGIST AND FERTILITY EXPERT

Sometimes menopause comes too soon, not because of the age you are when it occurs, but because it happens when you haven't yet completed your family. Conceiving a baby in menopause is not impossible, due to the occasional random burst of ovarian activity, but it is incredibly rare, and I have only seen it once in my entire career. But what about during perimenopause? Is it possible to consider being pregnant at that time? Well, it's not unheard of, however, but for most women, conceiving during perimenopause won't be as easy as becoming pregnant by accident, and you may need extra advice and help.

The perimenopause can last anywhere between 2 and 10 years and, whereas for the majority of women this starts in their 40s, it can begin much earlier (as discussed in the previous section). The consequences of this can be devastating and is the reason why fertility preservation, such as egg or embryo freezing, should always be considered where it's possible to anticipate an earlier menopause. The frozen egg or embryo can be stored until the point at which you might want to try to implant them.

Once you are perimenopausal, your chance of natural pregnancy is likely to be no more than around 2 per cent; even with IVF, if you use your own eggs, the success rate does not move past 5 per cent. However, egg donation significantly improves a woman's chances of conceiving to around 40 per cent. The statistics are incredibly discouraging and do not reflect the false impression created in the media about miracle babies being born to famous mothers in their 50s.

The reality is that almost all of these women will have used an egg donor, yet because there is still much taboo and stigma around this subject it isn't necessarily discussed openly with the public.

Egg donation, whereby another woman donates her eggs to you, can be the most wonderful and fulfilling experience, especially with new data from studies suggesting that the womb environment is able to affect the expression of donor genes, amplifying the bond between the carrier mother and child. However, the implications of having a child via this method are complex, and if you decide to go down this path, it's particularly important that you receive counselling to help you deal with this.

If using your own eggs, studies are showing us that positive lifestyle measures like good diet and exercise can significantly affect the health of those eggs and chance of implantation. Looking after yourself is the single best investment you can make in your, and your baby's, health.

'I think I've been living through it since I was about eight years old. A lot of great literature is based on the male menopause.'

ANDY HAMILTON, COMEDIAN AND CREATOR OF *DROP THE DEAD DONKEY*

SIXTEEN

Male menopause

expert view

LET'S TALK ABOUT . . . MALE MENOPAUSE

WITH PROFESSOR MALCOLM CARRUTHERS MD, SPECIALIST IN TESTOSTERONE DEFICIENCY

Men's testosterone levels start to fall naturally from their mid-20s onwards. These levels may be further depleted by stress, as well as poor diet or lifestyle choices and a number of other factors. By the time men hit the age of 50, our research at the Centre for Men's Health has shown that 20 per cent suffer from symptoms labelled as 'male menopause', 'andropause', or as it is more frequently termed these days, 'Testosterone Deficiency Syndrome'. However, despite its prevalence and the growing evidence to show that addressing men's testosterone needs is one of the most important areas of preventative medicine for the future, research shows only 1 percent of men are currently being treated for it under the NHS.

The effects of testosterone deficiency are usually more

gradual than those experienced by women during menopause, but the symptoms can be just as severe. Primarily, men usually experience difficulty in getting and maintaining an erection, and a particularly characteristic warning sign is losing morning erections, the 'morning glories'. This can be considered as the male equivalent of the loss of periods in women. Other symptoms include loss of sex drive (libido), irritability, depression, inability to concentrate, joint pains and even night sweats and hot flushes. There are a lot of similarities with the effects of menopause in women. These symptoms (in both sexes) can severely reduce enjoyment of life and love, and even cause relationships to break down.

HOW DO YOU KNOW IF YOU'RE AFFECTED?

Blood tests are offered, but the best way to diagnose any reduction in testosterone activity is a questionnaire called The Ageing Male Symptom Score (AMS). This asks men to grade, on a score from one to five, their experience of issues like: a decline in feelings of general wellbeing, joint pains, fall in muscular strength, decrease in beard growth and lowered libido. Given its usefulness we have made this available on the website for our clinic (**www.centreformenshealth.co.uk/mens-health-services/self-test-questionnaire**). Patients often report that getting their score from this was the lightbulb moment when they realised what might causing their symptoms.

At this point, a treatment called Testosterone Replacement Therapy (TRT), similar to the hormone replacement therapy used by women, can prevent and generally reverse the symptoms, but it's still not offered by many doctors. Conversely, at the Centre for Men's Health (Harley Street, London), we have made the diagnosis of andropause (and successfully and safely reversed its symptoms) in over 3,000 men using TRT.

Scare stories about the treatment causing prostate cancer or heart disease have been shown to be untrue. Testosterone treatment has proved to be both safe and effective, especially when given as a skin gel. However, I and other clinicians have documented what could be called 'hormonophobia' among other medics which prevents them using it.

This can happen for a number of reasons:

- *Failure to realise the urgency of the situation. Not understanding the severe impact that the combined symptomatology can have on the quality of life and the associated disease processes which may be starting due to hormone deficiencies.*
- *Lack of a true understanding of the safety of an increasing range of TRT and HRT preparations.*
- *Fears that have been generated by previous studies.*
- *Fears about the cost/benefits of different forms of TRT and HRT.*
- *Unwillingness to take responsibility for putting a man or woman on hormonal treatment and keeping them on it for several years or even using it as part of the basis of a health-promoting regime, for life.*

Because of 'hormonophobic' medics, the fate of the man who plucks up his courage to complain to his doctor of his menopause-like symptoms, or is urged by his partner to do so, is especially hard. He is told he is depressed, and treated with antidepressants, or given Viagra for his erection problems, which only works temporarily or not all, and doesn't solve the other emotional or physical symptoms. If he persists in thinking that his symptoms may be caused by low testosterone, he might be given a blood test, but while the NHS is become more open to the idea of testosterone deficiency (TD), it uses quite rigid and relatively low cut-offs on testosterone when deciding who to treat, rather than looking at symptoms. Many men are refused treatment on the basis that, despite having characteristic TD symptoms, their levels are 'normal' (even if low). These measures also don't rule out what's known as 'Low T-Activity' due to testosterone resistance. This is similar to the low insulin activity seen in diabetics due to insulin resistance where the body stops listening to testosterone's signals. The only true way to diagnose testosterone deficiency is therefore a recognition of the typical symptoms via the questionnaire and a trial of testosterone treatment to see if things improve.

So, what should a man do? Well, despite its limitations, the NHS is still a reasonable starting point as more GPs are becoming better informed on testosterone deficiency. It's a good idea to take the AMS test but also look at the British Society for Sexual Medicine guidelines on testosterone deficiency (**www.guidelines.co.uk/mens-health/bssm-guideline-on-adult-testosterone-deficiency/453888.article**) so you are informed as to what should be offered. If tests are offered but the doctor still can't or won't treat you, then you may need to seek out a private specialist in men's health, urology or endocrinology that also has experience in TRT treatment.

Ideally, one day we will have significantly better access to treatment for symptomatic men with low testosterone. I'd like to see us move to a similar, symptoms-focused, diagnostic model to that routinely used in identifying women who would benefit from HRT. It's natural for men's hormone levels and balance to change as they age. Where this has no health impact there is no need for treatment. However, where this change negatively impacts their health, wellbeing or relationships, a trial of testosterone replacement treatment (TRT) should be considered in the same way as HRT would be where a woman's health is being affected by the effects of menopause.

'I just want to raise awareness of the menopause in trans men – to make it easier to seek and get treatment.'

BUCK ANGEL, ACTOR, PRODUCER AND MOTIVATIONAL SPEAKER

SEVENTEEN

Trans menopause

My Story

A transgender person is a person who does not identify as the gender they were assigned at birth. I admit I hadn't really thought about their experience of the menopause until I spent time with a friend of mine, Buck Angel. Over 20 years ago, he transitioned and is affectionately known as 'Transpa', offering support and advice to many of the trans community.

Buck was assigned a female gender at birth, however, he identified as male from a young age. He chose to have his breasts removed but did not have a hysterectomy or have surgery below the waist. A female transitioning to male will often deal with menopausal symptoms sooner than anticipated as the hormone testosterone decreases the production of oestrogen.

I found it hard enough to get information on the menopause but advice and support as a transgender person is almost non-existent. Trying to get support for any gynaecological issues as a man is challenging. Going for smear tests, Buck found many gynaecologists refused to see him. We all know that the medical profession has limited knowledge about the menopause; for a trans man the knowledge is even more sparse. This makes me angry - comprehensive healthcare is the right of everyone. Every trans person should get the help they need to enjoy the life they want to be able to live.

There are also issues in other areas of life. Many workplaces now have supportive menopause policies, but many trans people don't want to (and shouldn't have to) disclose their status to their employers, which can make it difficult to take advantage of these policies. Negative attitudes from family and friends can add to the isolation.

So, with huge thanks at his openness and willingness to bring this topic into the open, I pass the rest of this chapter over to Buck, who has written his story for us to increase understanding and awareness. I hope it helps any transgender person reading, and perhaps educates some of the medical world too.

Buck's story

My name is Buck Angel. I am a transsexual man. I transitioned from a woman to a man over 23 years ago, with the use of testosterone, administered through a needle every week (and for the rest of my life).

This gave me the masculine appearance I have now and after about two years on testosterone, I then proceeded to remove my breasts surgically to give me a male chest. During this time in my transition, I desired a penis. This was not an easy surgeon to find; there were very little transgender resources back then and the internet was barely available. I eventually opted out of getting the penis surgery as I did not feel confident it was the right choice considering the lack of information.

So, I kept my vagina and I had to teach myself how to walk the world as a man with a vagina – before most people even knew what transgender was. I eventually became known as the man with a vagina. As I grew into my transition, aches and pains came. On some level, I was an experiment. Unlike today where there is a growing trans community willing to speak about their experiences, there were not many guys before me who were public about transitioning, and there was little, if any, knowledge on long-term use of testosterone on a female-bodied person.

One of the most dramatic changes that happen with transgender men is to your physical appearance due to the reduction of oestrogen when testosterone becomes your prominent hormone. Body hair grows, muscles come, your voice changes and even your facial features begin to become more masculine. I even lost the hair on my head! But as this happens outside there are also changes within the body that you can't see with the naked eye, and I had no idea what was about to happen to my body.

After about 10 years on testosterone, I started getting very bad cramping in my pelvic area. Specifically, right after sex, it felt just like period cramps but without blood. Sometimes these cramps would go on for hours and have me doubled over in pain. I would seek advice from gynaecologists only to either be told that they could not see me because they were uncomfortable with my kind, or they would give me a pap smear and tell me everything was ok and that the cramps were normal. This went on for years and years.

Eventually, I moved out of the USA to live in Yucatán, Mexico. In Mexico, no one knew I used to be a woman, so when I dropped on the floor one day with a temperature of 40.5°C, I was taken to the emergency room. The doctors rushed to me, and I told them I was a transsexual because I knew they would be taking my clothes off. The doctors told me to calm down as I was septic, and they were trying to figure it out. Had I come in five minutes later, I would have died.

With tests, they realised the issue, and for the first time someone knew what was happening with my body. They told me that the long-

term use of testosterone had atrophied my reproductive system causing my uterus to fuse with my cervix, creating an infection in my uterus. That was the cramping I had been experiencing all these years.

Now, my uterus had burst, causing the infection to enter the bloodstream and causing me to become septic. The doctor told me I had atrophied. I had never heard the word before and had no idea what it even meant, but they told me that in order for a vagina to function it needs oestrogen. The testosterone I had been injecting removed my oestrogen; I would have been fine if I had also been using a low-dose oestrogen supplement. I was never ever told this by any doctor in the USA. Ever.

After three months on intensive antibiotics to get rid of the infection, I then had a full laparoscopic vaginal hysterectomy. The doctors in Mexico who performed this said they had never seen a reproductive system so atrophied.

All of this could have been prevented if any one of my endocrinologists would have given me an oestrogen supplement. This is why I am now a voice in the transgender male community on vaginal wellness. How can doctors be giving a very powerful hormone-like testosterone without understanding the need to balance this out? Is it because it deals with the vagina and not the penis? Is it because we do not care about vaginal health for women or men?

Today, we have a responsibility to discuss these important health concerns for anyone with a vagina. I almost died because of the lack of medical knowledge, yet the doctors give testosterone out with little concern about the long-term effects. The last thing I want to see is a trans man having to deal with the same life-threatening situation I did, just because they want to live fully and authentically as a man.

expert view

LET'S TALK ABOUT . . . TRANS MENOPAUSE

WITH DR RIXT LUIKENAAR, GYNAECOLOGIST

The experience of menopause differs greatly among transgender men. Transgender men who undergo hysterectomy and have their ovaries removed will go through surgical menopause at the time of surgery. Talking to them about their experience of menopausal hot flushes after surgery reveals that many don't notice them at all, some have a few hot flushes, and others notice symptoms a few years after their surgery. The testosterone seems to be overbearing for transgender men in contrary to cisgender women who experience significant menopausal symptoms after surgical menopause.

We are not sure of the long-term effects of ovary removal in transgender men on testosterone as we don't have enough data from studies of those using testosterone over 10, 20, and 30 years to form a clear picture. We suspect that, as in cisgender women, the loss of oestrogen can lead to long-term health problems but external testosterone supplementation may prevent this.

When I counsel my patients during transition, I have a conversation with them about what hormones are and what they do, and I explain that if I remove their ovaries they will have no oestrogen and they will go into menopause. Some are so young, just in their 20s, and I explain that oestrogen offers protective benefits in regards to bone density, heart and brain health and potentially other conditions. Removing this now means they have to be extremely careful to protect their bones, and look after their heart, by living a healthy lifestyle, taking vitamin D3, eating calcium-rich products and engaging in weight-bearing exercise their entire life. I therefore suggest that perhaps they hang on to their ovaries for 10–20 years so they at least get that protection (and for fertility preservation). Some agree, others don't feel that they want them in their body any longer as it feels foreign, or they don't want the risk for ovarian cancer or to deal with PMS.

Transgender men who haven't had their ovaries removed during transition still produce oestrogen and eggs, even in the presence of testosterone. They go through natural menopause in their late 40s and 50s but also often don't notice the typical symptoms of menopause.

However, one thing both groups may experience is vaginal atrophy or vaginal dryness. This can be treated with a local oestrogen cream. which doesn't interfere with testosterone production. In some cases. though, not only do the tissues of the vagina become really thin, red and irritated, they also develop a discharge that almost looks like glue – and it sticks like glue (desquamous vaginitis). Internally, it can glue the ovaries, tubes, uterus and the bowel together and it causes significant pelvic pain. This is similar to what happens in endometriosis, but it doesn't look exactly the same during laparoscopy. This is what happened to Buck, and I've operated on about five other men who have had severe pelvic pain and cramping and found the same findings inside their abdomen. We don't think it's caused by a decrease in oestrogen, but from a reaction to the use of testosterone. It doesn't happen to every transgender man, but it can happen.

For this and other reasons, transgender men need to have gynaecological check-ups (even after a hysterectomy). You need to be investigated if you develop unusual discharge, pain or bleeding. You also need screening smear tests if you have a cervix. Gynaecological conditions such as vulval cancer, HPV and sexual transmitted diseases can happen to all cisgender women and transgender men.

The good news is there are more gynaecologists becoming aware of the need for this care. To find someone specialising in this area, you may need to speak to other trans men, contact LGBTQ healthcare centres in your areas, or contact the World Professional Association for Transgender Health WPATH (www.wpath.org) who might be able to help, but it's important you consider it as part of your medical care.

“

‘One thing both groups may experience is vaginal atrophy or vaginal dryness. This can be treated with a local oestrogen cream which doesn’t interfere with testosterone production.’

'Now I am a menopausal Mama, I am having the time of my life. I am doing a lot more adventurous stuff… It's a very free time in my life.'

CAROL VORDERMAN,
TV PRESENTER

EIGHTEEN

A Charge for the better

My Story

When I started the menopause, I thought it was the beginning of the end. Happier and more content than ever, I now know I was very wrong. It was challenging at times, but I paid my dues and am now reaping the benefits of being older and more comfortable with who I am.

Society seems to assign us all to the scrapheap when we hit a certain age and assume that our lives are downhill from there. Remain young and fertile if you want to be useful, seems to be the media refrain. The pressure is crippling, and I want to shift that narrative, so all women move from a feeling of weakness to a feeling of empowerment as they approach their second spring.

No more periods and spending money on tampons is just one benefit. Embracing life and exploring new avenues in this stage of life is an incredible experience, and I intend to make the most of every moment. Jennifer Aniston, Courtney Cox, Andrea McLean, Jennifer Lopez, Davina McCall, Carol Vorderman and so many more, are all rewriting the script on what it means to be middle-aged. Reaching this age is a privilege denied to many, and if all our sisters who we've loved and lost were able to talk to us then I am sure they would tell us just to 'go for it' and have as many 'fuck it' moments as we can.

'Fuck it' moments are my version of the 'bucket list', I have taken out a new membership to living, and these moments are amongst the many benefits. Over the last couple of years, I have overcome extreme anxiety to talk at events about the menopause; present my own podcast; write for many magazines; appear on many TV shows; and develop a menopausal product range. I feel I have a purpose now. This was unthinkable in my 40s, when fear of failure and what people might think would have held me back. I don't care as much now if I mess up. People who matter won't judge me, and the people who do judge me – well, that's their problem. I've dropped the people-pleasing that I was so guilty of, and now spend time with people that celebrate me, not tolerate me.

I love piercings and now have 29 of them. Some may judge me, but I don't care – I love them! When I turned 50 I had a tattoo of a little heart on my face and had 'this too shall pass' inked on my chest as a reminder that things do get better. I also had 'love yourself first' inked on my arm as a reminder to practise self-compassion. Again, some may think I have lost the plot – but I don't care. I love my piercings and tattoos – and may well have more. There will always be a bit of rebel inside me.

Envying others is another emotion I have happily said goodbye to. I used to think the grass was always greener elsewhere. I know now that the grass is just fine where I am. And if it isn't – well, it's up to me to sort my garden out. My ego is so much stronger; if there is a bad story in the press or an awful photo, I can just brush it off. I have stopped giving power to others.

I have absolutely no intention of stopping – I certainly didn't get the memo that post-50 it is all over. I am looking into getting a pilot's licence and am excited about it. For someone who used to have a terror of driving, that is a huge thing for me. Exploring the possibility of living outside London is another big one; I love London but now wonder if I might love somewhere else just as much. Travelling more is also on the agenda. I am in discussions about documentaries and even thinking of taking a show to the Edinburgh Fringe. I am having more fun now than I ever did as a party girl!

Lobbying the government for more trained menopause nurse practitioners is also on my to-do list. My daughter's generation should not have to beg for help from their GP, so I am campaigning for exactly that. Menopause in the storylines of soaps is another thing I want to see, so it is in the front rooms of households everywhere. I keep an eye out for opportunities, so please get in touch on my social - media platforms if you have any ideas. My team is open to helping wherever possible – finding experts and basically breaking and battering down doors to make things happen.

So how can you embrace this same menopause positivity? Over to Lorraine Candy, an amazing journalist whose attitude to life after menopause I absolutely love, for her advice.

expert view

LET'S TALK ABOUT . . . THE NEW MENOPAUSE POSITIVITY

WITH LORRAINE CANDY, JOURNALIST

My menopause came with no warning, no reference points, no cultural signposts. One day I was fine, the next I wasn't. After a successful media career travelling the world and a decade of amazing, but busy, mothering of four kids, I expected, in my fifth decade, to enter a new phase of strength, confident in the world around me... instead I was a mess.

Now I am in a much happier, more positive, and indeed more powerful place, and I can tell you that if you feel like I did, you will come out of the dark and into the light but you must ask for help.

My menopause was an unhappy time because I kept it a secret, but you should talk about your experience to others. Now, on the other side, I think I am a smarter, bolder version of myself. The fog has lifted. The happy times are here. But should you still be in that gloomy, panic-inducing, sad and often hopeless place I was, then I have some words of wisdom for you:

LEARN TO SINGLE TASK

Stop doing two or three things at the same time; it's kinder on yourself. Once you start this, you realise it is the path to a more peaceful mind, which is a powerful feeling. It's possible. I have done it. Start to notice when you do too many things and stop them all bar one; I promise no one will die. It will be fine.

YOU MAY NOT FEEL SEXY BUT TRUST ME YOU ARE

You haven't lost this part of you, it's just changed and you've got at least 30 years to explore new pleasures. I was furious that I was too old to justify a second glance from men in the street (inexplicable I know) because I thought my attractiveness was attached to my looks. It's not, it never was; this realisation is like getting a superpower. Relish it.

FIND YOUR FRIENDS

Prune out the ones who don't make you happy, love the ones who do, and make time to see them and find new ones. The girlfriends I have made in the past two years have changed my outlook completely. I am so glad I was open to them and made an effort to keep them close.

TUNE INTO YOUR NEWLY DEVELOPED BULLSHIT COUNTER

You have life experience. Your instinct is now always right about the people, the places, the jobs, the situations you think reek of wrongness. Step away from them. This is actually your brain working like a computer, not a gut feeling – it's seen it before. Your internal algorithm has kicked in. Just say 'No'.

REMEMBER THAT EXPERIENCE, NOT STUFF, MATTERS

My hard-earned money goes on memories now, not things.

> ***'Menopause has been the hardest part of my life, but it has given me a renewed determination to enjoy the rest of my life now that I am well.'***

CALM DOWN

Who cares what people think of you? Not everyone can like you; it's statistics and nothing to do with who you actually are. Being this way becomes easier in your 50s. You lose any defensiveness you had, you are able to shrug your shoulders, because you can choose if today is going to be a good day or not; you can choose how you handle it and who you ask for help.

TAKE UP A NEW HOBBY

I found open water swimming. I learnt front crawl and met a group of people all round the country who have made me laugh, made me happy and made me cake. Find your 'swimming', it will change your life.

And that's it, really. So much to look forward to. So many lovely, new happy times ahead. It's like a new beginning but even better.

MENOPAUSE IN THE FUTURE

I've talked a lot in this book about how menopause has been dealt with in the past and what we need to change now to make things better – but what might happen with the treatment of menopause in the future?

Actually, quite a lot. It seems like scientists are as keen as we are to make this process easier, and they are working on a lot of different drugs and other treatments to help relieve symptoms for those who can't use HRT, or would prefer not to. Most promising, according to my science gurus, is a drug that has been used to treat a problem called polycystic ovary syndrome, but that has also been found to reduce the effects of hot flushes, weight gain, poor sleeping and poor concentration in menopause. It's being created in London and if all goes well, might be on the market around 2021.

There's also a huge wave toward menopause gizmos – 'meno-tech'. As I write this, there's a couple of cooling devices being invented that should be on the market very soon, including one that you can pop out of your handbag and hold to cool yourself down when a flush comes. More innovations into cooling nightwear and bedclothes are on their way, and there are even apps coming out that use CBT techniques to help you handle flushes by focusing on snowy scenes.

Lastly, way off into the future, women might be able to choose when to have their menopause. A treatment called ovary grafting sees a small piece of tissue removed from the ovaries. This tissue contains eggs and can produce oestrogen. It would be removed when women are young, stored until around the age of menopause, then added back to the ovary where it can take over some of the work from the older ovary. If the tissue is removed from a 20-something, the scientists say it could delay menopause for 20 years. Taken from a 40-something, it might hold things back for five years. It's already available privately to women under 40 as a treatment for early menopause in one clinic in England, but the doctors say it has the potential in the future to be used on any woman who wants to delay menopause for a while.

Another treatment is using parts of plasma (a fluid found in blood) to wake up the ovaries and make them act younger again, while doctors in the US are creating artificial ovaries that, if it all goes as planned, could be put into the body to take over the job of your own ovaries, stopping menopause completely. The downside of this is that it does mean you might still have periods and the possibility of getting pregnant at 70!

What it goes to show is that things are changing all the time in the menopause world. To keep up to date, I would recommend:

- **My Instagram account:** MegsMenopause
- **My website:** megsmenopause.com
- **My podcast:** Megs Menopause
- **The NHS official website:** www.nhs.uk – and search for menopause
- **Dr Louise Newson's excellent website:** menopausedoctor.co.uk
- **Keep updated on the NICE Guidelines:** www.nice.org.uk
- **The British Menopausal Society:** www.thebms.org.uk

afterword

THANKS, MENOPAUSE, I OWE YOU ONE

And so we reach the last chapter. And, despite what you might think reading what I went through, I'd like to end the book by saying thanks to my menopause. I owe it a lot.

When my symptoms were at their worst, I remember one question circling my mind over and over again: how long is this going to last? But now, I appreciate what happened. It's given me the chance to find myself, who I was supposed to be. If I'd sailed through menopause, would that have happened? I don't know. Now, though, I have a purpose, and that's to help other women. I've gone from ripping up the London social scene to working hard on MegsMenopause and now I'm on a mission to make sure that other women know what to expect during menopause and that they have a community to lean on during the tough parts. And I love it… I feel that I have finally become the person I was always meant to be.

Every day, I wake up and go straight onto Instagram and answer questions, put out a post, have a chat with the women on there and I just feel fulfilled. They might be really simple questions, but knowing that I'm helping someone feel supported and that they are not on their own is such a great thing. My whole story now comes because of what happened to me and I wouldn't have understood that if I'd just read about menopause. I had to go through it and feel dreadful, and hate every second of it, so thanks, menopause, you really did change my life. You empowered me, you gave me confidence, you helped me cut through the bullshit and after years of living for other people, I am now living for me. And it feels bloody fantastic. So, it's time to sign off and I want to do it with a final word from Mary Portas, retail expert, broadcaster, founder of Work Like a Woman, and a woman I really admire in many areas of life - including how she sees menopause. I hope this and the rest of the book gives you a new understanding and feeling of control on what's happening now, and a new hope for what happens next. Trust me, menos - it rocks on this side of the fence.

A FINAL WORD

BY MARY PORTAS

As mid-life women, we have something in common with one of the most powerful and majestic creatures of the sea - the killer whale. They are the only other species to go through menopause. But, unlike many other species (including humans), they are not then deemed invisible and of limited use. They take on a leadership role, using their experience to locate salmon to feed the pod and younger orcas stay by her side, recognising her as the wise elder from whom they can learn so much.

Like the killer whale, I challenge society's negative narrative around getting older. Life excites me, and there is so much still to discover. Women in their 50s, 60s, 70s and beyond, are breaking out of comfort zones to move into unchartered waters, finding it sometimes scary, but always exhilarating. They are moving into new careers, travelling to new countries, starting up new businesses, beginning new relationships, and exploring their creativity in new ventures. Listening carefully to their feelings and paying attention to what makes them feel energised, connected and stimulated, they are then giving those things the oxygen they need to thrive.

Looking back, I think I truly got into my stride around the age of 46 when I was perimenopausal. I stopped editing myself to suit other's expectations and started presenting myself filter-free. What I wear and what I do reflects me – colourful, confident and slightly flamboyant. Like so many others, I wasted time complying with other people's ideas of who I should be. I am not integrating into society's norms; I am planting my own garden and watching it bloom. Not everyone likes it, but I no longer afford them the power to influence how I live. The joy of being completely true to yourself is like feeling the warm glow you get from a couple of glasses of good wine. It's like hearing the radio station you love clear as a bell after spending time trying to tune it in and hearing only buzzing and hissing.

Transformation has always thrilled me – of stores, high streets, home interiors and fashion trends. People also fascinate me, so watching people transform themselves is particularly intriguing for me. As we get older, I see so many women change from the person they thought they had to be and become who they were always meant to be. It's like a light has been switched on within them. Even if some of the ventures don't work, we can always try again or simply try something new. I am a big fan of JFDI - Just F***ing Do It. Remember learning to ride a bike? When you fell off the first time, you probably didn't give up and say 'oh well, clearly this bike riding isn't for me' - you kept on trying until all of a sudden you were hurtling down hills with your hands in the air. And if you really didn't like it or take to it - you got out roller skates or a scooter or tried something different. Recapturing that childlike approach to life and experiencing the thrill of trying the new and unfamiliar leads to surges in energy and true joy in living.

I want this book to give you hope that you are simply moving to a new stage in life. A time for introspection on what makes you totally, truly and completely happy. A time to leave the crap behind, to eliminate anything that you feel is not connected to your true self, so that you can have the time for what really makes your soul sing. We have spent a fair few decades building life experience, emotional intelligence and a sense of who we are - this time is when all that investment pays off.

We all have a natural energy and sensitivity as women, which traditionally we may have felt a need to suppress. Things are changing now and the values that I respect in women (and many men) that are considered feminine, are increasing in value in society - both in and out of the workplace. Kindness, life ambition, and working with instinct, are examples of such traits that are increasingly regarded in a positive light. You are never too old - and it is never too late - to start pursuing your most authentic self.

So, be inspired by the killer whale and step up to the life you deserve with self-confidence and the knowledge that you are enough.

Appendix A

MEG'S MENO-DICTIONARY

This is a list of words and terms we use in the book, or that you might come across elsewhere in your menopause journey that you might not have heard before. Here's what they mean:

ADHD: Stands for Attention Deficit Hyperactivity Disorder. Symptoms include impulsivity, short attention span and hyperactivity.

ADRENALS: Small glands located on top of each kidney. They produce stress hormones like cortisol and adrenaline. They also produce weak androgens.

ANDROGENS: Male sex hormones including testosterone. Even women produce low levels of these.

ANDROPAUSE: The medical term for male menopause. Commonly linked to a fall in testosterone.

BIOIDENTICAL HORMONES: Manufactured versions of oestrogen, progesterone and testosterone that are identical in structure to the hormones made by your own body. Often made from plants like yams and soy.

BODY IDENTICAL HORMONES: Usually refers to regulated forms of bioidentical hormones. May also be referred to as rBHRT – Regulated Bioidentical Hormone Replacement Therapy.

BONE DENSITY: A measure of how thick and dense the bones are. Low bone density is a signof osteoporosis.

BULLET VIBRATOR: A vibrating sex toy, kind of shaped like a bullet.

CARDIOVASCULAR DISEASE: Diseases of the heart and blood vessels, like coronary heart disease, stroke or peripheral artery disease.

CATASTROPHISING: Away of thinking where you think the worst-case scenario.

CBD OIL: Oil containing cannabidiol - an ingredient found in plants of the cannabis family.

CISGENDER: A person whose gender identifies with the sex they were assigned at birth.

CLITORAL HOOD: Fold of skin that covers the clitoris, protecting it from irritation.

COGNITIVE BEHAVIOUR THERAPY: Also known as CBT, this is a talking therapy that aims to help you change your beliefs about things, which then also helps change your behaviour.

COMPOUNDED BIOIDENTICAL HORMONES: Bioidentical hormones made in compounding pharmacies to your unique prescription. They may also include other hormones like DHEA and androstenedione that are not regulated for use in the UK. Sometimes called cBHRT by medical professionals.

CONTINUOUS COMBINATION THERAPY: A form of HRT where you take both oestrogen and progesterone every day of the month.

DEEP VEIN THROMBOSIS: A blood clot that forms in the deep veins of the body like those in the leg.

DEXA SCAN: An imaging test that checks for bone density. Used to help spot osteoporosis.

DILATOR: A device you can

insert into the vagina to gently stretch the walls to get you used to penetration.

DONOR EGGS: Eggs donated by another woman to be used in fertility treatment.

EARLY OVARIAN AGEING: Reduced function of the ovaries - i.e, producing less oestrogen and not releasing eggs every month - for your age. You can still be fertile with EOA and have periods but it can progress to early menopause.

EARLY MENOPAUSE: Defined as when periods stop before the age of 40.

EGG FREEZING: Technique used to preserve fertility where eggs are removed from the ovaries and stored.

EMBRYO FREEZING: A step on from egg freezing; the egg is fertilised with sperm and the resulting embryos are stored.

ENDOCRINOLOGY: The area of medicine involving hormones.

EPISIOTOMY: Cut made at the edge of the vagina during childbirth to help deliver the baby.

FSH TEST: Measures level of follicle stimulating hormone. If these are high it can signify that you are in, or approaching, menopause. Usually only used to detect early or premature menopause.

GENITOURINARY: Issues that include the genitals and/or the urinary system.

GERIATRIC PREGNANCY: The medical term for having a baby past the age of 35.

HORMONE REPLACEMENT THERAPY: The use of oestrogen - and sometimes progesterone - to replace the hormones that fall during perimenopause and menopause.

HYSTERECTOMY: Surgical removal of the uterus (womb). May also involve the removal of the ovaries, fallopian tube and/or cervix.

INFLAMMATION: The system the body uses to protect itself against infection. It's natural, but long-lasting inflammation can be detrimental to health.

ISOFLAVONES: Ingredients in some foods that act like oestrogen in the body. They are part of the group of substances called phytoestrogens.

IVF: In Vitro Fertilisation. A treatment that can be used when conception isn't happening naturally. Doctors fertilise an egg outside the womb and the embryo is put back into the woman to develop.

LIBIDO: The desire for sexual activity.

LICHEN SCLEROSIS: Condition that can affect the skin of the vulva. It causes a white shiny appearance to the skin and itching.

MBSR: Mindfulness-based stress reduction. Uses mindfulness – the art of living in the now rather than focusing on the past or future – to help reduce stress and anxiety.

MEDICAL MENOPAUSE: Also known as induced menopause, this is menopause triggered by medical treatment that damages the ovaries.

MENOPAUSE: The point when periods permanently stop. To have officially reached menopause, your periods need to have stopped for 12 months.

MICRONISED PROGESTERONE: A form of progesterone made from plants used in HRT.

NICE GUIDELINES: NICE stands for the National Institute of Clinical Excellence. This medical body decides the best practice for how conditions should be treated in the UK. These are called NICE Guidelines.

OESTROGEN: Female hormone secreted by the ovaries.

OESTROGEN PESSARY: Form of oestrogen delivered through the vagina.

OOPHORECTOMY: Removal of an ovary or ovaries.

OSTEOPOROSIS: Medical condition where the bones become thin and brittle with increased risk of fracture.

OVARIES: Part of the female reproductive system in which eggs are produced.

PEEZE: Meg's word for when you pee when you sneeze.

PELVIC FLOOR: The layer of muscles that support the bowels, bladder and vagina.

PERIMENOPAUSE: The time leading up to the menopause. It can start up to ten years before the periods actually stop.

PHYTOESTROGENS: Naturally occurring substances in foods like soy that act the same way as oestrogens in the body.

POST-MENOPAUSE: You are classed as in post-menopause one year after your periods stop completely.

PREMATURE MENOPAUSE: In the UK, this is another term for early menopause. In some other countries it specifically means the cessation of periods after 40 but before the age of 45.

PREMATURE OVARIAN INSUFFICIENCY: Another phrase for early or premature menopause.

PROGESTERONE: Female hormone secreted by the ovaries.

PROGESTOGEN: A synthetic hormone that acts in the same way as progesterone.

PSYCHOSEXUAL: The mental and emotional side of sexual activity.

RESISTANCE TRAINING: Types of exercise that use pressure on the muscles to strengthen them – weight training is a good example, but so are moves like press ups and squats.

SEROTONIN: Chemical produced in the brain that's involved with mood.

SEQUENTIAL COMBINATION THERAPY: HRT regime where you take oestrogen all month, but only use progesterone for 10–14 days every month, or every three months. Also known as cyclical HRT.

SMEAR TEST: Test to check for any change or abnormalities in the cells of the cervix that may lead to cervical cancer.

STRESS INCONTINENCE: Leaking urine when you cough, sneeze, run or do other sudden movements. Caused by a weak pelvic floor.

SURGICAL MENOPAUSE: Menopause brought on by the surgical removal of the ovaries.

TESTOSTERONE: One of the androgens - or male-type - hormones. Women have low levels of this produced by the ovaries and adrenal glands.

TRANSDERMAL: Delivered through the skin.

TRANSGENDER: Person whose sense of gender identify does not correspond with the sex they were assigned at birth.

VAGINA: The internal part of your genitals; it's a muscular tube that runs from the vaginal opening up to the cervix.

VAGINAL ATROPHY: Thinning of the walls of the vagina caused by falling oestrogen levels.

VAGINAL REJUVENATION: Surgery or laser treatment to improve the appearance, tone and health of the vagina and vaginal tissues.

VULVA: The external part of female genitals. It includes the labia minora, the labia majora and the clitoris.

Appendix B

WHO'S WHO

So many people helped me with this book and I can't thank them enough – here's more detail on all of them and how you can find out more about them.

MS TANIA ADIB

MD MRCOG

Former Lead Clinician for Colposcopy and Lead Clinician for Gynaecological Oncology at the Queen's Hospital in London. She also works at many other London health clinics. You can see more about her work at **www.adib.org.uk**.

BUCK ANGEL

An entrepreneur in the field of transgender sexual health and a transgender activist. Buck was born female on 5 June 1962. He never felt female and struggled through life until he had the life-changing opportunity to transition from female to male and finally live life authentically. He now inspires and educates an entire generation on the fluidity of sexuality and identity politics.

DR MEG ARROLL

PhD, CPsychol, CSci, AFBPsS, FHEA, MISCPAccred

A chartered psychologist and scientist based in Harley Street, London. She is also author of six health books. Find out more about her or contact her via **www.drmegarroll.com**.

DAWN BRESLIN

TV and radio presenter, Dawn is a bestselling author and the founder of the Harmonizing Academy. She has inspired thousands of women to heal, re-energise and transform their lives. **https://dawnbreslin.com**.

LORRAINE CANDY
Journalist and editor at the *Sunday Times* as luxury content director and editor-in-chief of the *Sunday Times Style* magazine. She also writes a weekly family column for the *Sunday Times* magazine.

PROFESSOR MALCOLM CARRUTHERS
Founder of the Centre for Men's Health in Harley Street, London. He is a highly respected men's health specialist and world authority on testosterone deficiency. Find out more in his book *The 50+Plan: His and Hers HRT* (The Andropause Society) and on the website **www.centreformenshealth.co.uk**.

DR LARISA CORDA
MBBS BSc MRCOG
A women's health expert and fertility expert working in London and pioneer of a unique holistic approach to fertility and pregnancy called The Conception Plan, as featured on This Morning. Learn more about her work at **www.drlarisacorda.com**.

DIANE DANZEBRINK
Private therapist to women and couples and wellbeing consultant to businesses and organisations. She is the founder of **www.menopausesupport.co.uk** and the #MakeMenopauseMatter campaign which is calling for major improvements in menopause care and support. **www.dianedanzebrink.com**.

LIZ EARLE MBE
Founder of **www.lizearlewellbeing.com**. Liz has been a respected and award-winning authority in the world of beauty, natural nutrition and wellbeing for over 30 years.

LYNNE FRANKS
Founder of SEED. Go to **www.lynnefranks.com** and **www.hubatno3.com**.

ANAÏS GALLAGHER
Model and photographer and online contributing editor to *Tatler*.

CAROLINE GASKIN

MCPH

First started studying homeopathy in 1994 and is now one of the UK's most well-respected homeopathic and natural practitioners. She runs numerous workshops and retreats in the UK and around the world. See more on her website **www.carolinegaskin.co.uk**.

SARAH GRANT

BANT CNCH

Nutritional therapist and health coach who works in London. She specialises in the interaction between the health of the gut and the health of the body. See more at **www.gutreaction.co.uk**.

BETHANY HARROLD

Experienced early menopause at 15. She now works at The Daisy Network as Social-Media Manager and runs a non-profit organisation called The Fabulous Fertility Fundraiser, raising awareness and holding events to fundraise for UK charities surrounding infertility, adoption and child-loss.

MISS ANNE HENDERSON

MA MB BChir MA MRCOG

A highly experienced Consultant Obstetrician and Gynaecologist working in Kent and Harley Street, London. She is also a British Menopause Society Accredited specialist, a recognition which is applied to only 150 consultants in the UK. See more at **www.gynae-expert.co.uk**.

AILSA HICHENS

ANT CNHC

Registered Nutritional Therapist and health coach for women whose hormones are a little out of balance. She practises in Chelmsford, Essex. See more at **www.foodfabulous.co.uk**.

ROB HOBSON

MSC

Registered nutritionist (Association for Nutrition). He has worked with celebrities, many of the UK's largest food and health companies, and the NHS for over a decade. See more about him at **www.robhobson.co.uk.**

CHRISTINA HOWELLS

BSC MSC

London-based personal trainer with over 25 years of experience. She has an Exercise and Sport Science BSc Hons and an MSc in Sport and Exercise Psychology. See more about her at **www.thatgirllondon.com**.

DR LAURA JARVIS

MBCHB, DRCOG, DFFP, MIPM

A specialty doctor in Sexual and Reproductive Health in Tayside. She is also a member of the Institute of Psychosexual Medicine and a menopause specialist. Follow her on twitter @LauraJa70798432.

ANABEL KINGSLEY

Consultant Trichologist. She works at the Philip Kingsley clinics, set up by her late father, the renowned trichologist Philip Kingsley. See more at **www.philipkingsley.co.uk**.

JANE LEWIS

Campaigner about vaginal atrophy to bring awareness about the condition. Over the past few years she has given talks, created social media groups and written a book: *Me and My Menopausal vagina: Living With Vaginal Atrophy* (PAL Books).

DR RIXT LUIKENAAR

Obstetrician and gynaecologist who works in Salt Lake City, Utah. She works with many trans patients and has won numerous awards for her education work in this field. See more at **www.rebirthobgyn.com**.

ELAINE MILLER

Fellow of the Chartered Society of Physiotherapy. She's also a comedian, mother of three and a recovered incontinent. She is passionate about leaky ladies, uses humour to break down taboos, and wants you to #laughnotleak.

DR LOUISE NEWSON

BSc (Hons) MB ChB (Hons) MRCP FRCGP

GP and menopause expert based at the Newson Health Menopause and Wellbeing Centre in Stratford-upon-Avon. Her menopause website is **www.menopause doctor.co.uk**. Information about her app, Balance, is available at balance-app.com.

MARY PORTAS

Retail expert, passionate about making Britain's shops better businesses and its people better consumers. She is campaigning for rights of women in the workplace via her latest initiative Work Like a Woman. She has also presented many radio and television programmes on business and retail.

CLARE PRENDERGAST

BA Hons, PGCE, PG Dip

Relationship and Psychosexual Therapist practising in Manchester. She is an accredited member of the College of Sexual and Relationship Therapists. See more at **www.manchestertherapist.co.uk**.

DR BELLA SMITH

MBBS BMedSci, MRCP MRCGP, FSRH

GP with an interest in women's health based in Suffolk, and a GP advisor for The Eve Appeal, a UK-based gynaecological cancer charity. She is also founder of @theDigitalGp.

DR NIGMA TALIB

ND

Board-certified Naturopathic doctor. She is based in Los Angeles where she works with some of the world's most famous and beautiful women. See more about her approach in her book, *Reverse the Signs of Ageing* (Vermilion) or on her website **www.healthydoc.com**.

LUCY WYNDHAM-READ

Women's fitness expert and author of the *7-Minute Body Plan* (Dorling Kindersley). Check out her Instagram for more fitness **@lucywyndhamread**.

JO WOOD

Model, television personality and entrepreneur.

THANK YOU TO:

Everyone who keeps me sober.

Janice Vee, for sharing my menopause journey in the first years of not knowing.

Sarah Bailey for making me career-shifter of the year at *Red* magazine and giving me a column on the menopause.

Jennifer Kennedy and Helen Foster for coming to my rescue and helping deliver this book.

Dr Sara Matthews.

Dr Louise Newson.

Dr Shahzadi Harper.

NHS Chelsea and Westminster Menopause Clinic.

Everyone at the NHS Adelaide Health Surgery.

And last but not least – the invention of the Box Set/ Netflix/Apple TV/Now TV!!

INDEX

MM indicates Meg Mathews.
Page references in *italics* indicate images.

SYMPTOM INDEX

3

Vermilion, an imprint of Ebury Publishing,
20 Vauxhall Bridge Road,
London, SW1V 2SA

Vermilion is part of the Penguin Random House group of companies whose addresses can be found at global.penguinrandomhouse.com

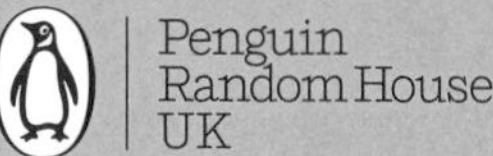

First published by Vermilion in 2020

www.penguin.co.uk

A CIP catalogue record for this book is available from the British Library

Design: Nikki Dupin at Studio Nic & Lou
Illustration: Adelaide Leeder

ISBN: 9781785042539

Printed and bound in Latvia by Livonia Print

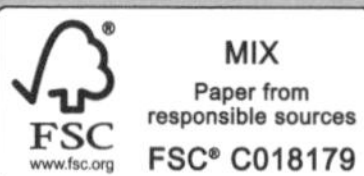

Penguin Random House is committed to a sustainable future for our business, our readers and our planet. This book is made from Forest Stewardship Council® certified paper.